NEUROLOGICAL
DRUG
REACTIONS AND
INTERACTIONS

NEUROLOGICAL
DRUG
REACTIONS AND
INTERACTIONS

JEROME Z. LITT, MD

Assistant Clinical Professor of Dermatology
Case Western Reserve University School of Medicine
Cleveland, Ohio

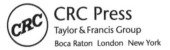

CRC Press
Taylor & Francis Group
Boca Raton London New York

CRC Press is an imprint of the
Taylor & Francis Group, an **informa** business

CRC Press
Taylor & Francis Group
6000 Broken Sound Parkway NW, Suite 300
Boca Raton, FL 33487-2742

Visit the Taylor & Francis Web site at
http://www.taylorandfrancis.com

and the CRC Press Web site at
http://www.crcpress.com

CONTENTS

INTRODUCTION

Any drug can cause any rash.

According to the World Health Organization, an adverse reaction (ADR) – or adverse event (ADE) – to a drug has been defined as any noxious or unintended reaction to a drug that has been administered in standard doses by the proper route for the purposes of prophylaxis, diagnosis, or treatment. This definition does not include abuse, overdose, withdrawal, or error of administration. While most reactions are mild and self-limited, severe and life-threatening reactions do occur, as seen in Coma and Stroke. Death is the ultimate adverse drug event, and has now been incorporated into the book.

ADRs are underreported and thus are an underestimated cause of morbidity and mortality. The incidence and severity of ADRs can be influenced by age, sex, disease, genetic factors, type of drug, route of administration, duration of therapy, dosage, and bioavailability, as well as interactions with other drugs. It has been estimated that fatal ADRs are the third or fourth leading cause of death in the US.

This pocketbook of Neurological Drug Reactions and Interactions describes and catalogs the adverse effects of over 260 commonly prescribed and over-the-counter generic drugs and herbals used in neurology or having neurological side effects. These drugs include classes such as Anticholinergic agents, Anticonvulsants, Antimigraine agents, Anti-Parkinsonian agents and Neuromuscular blockers. The drugs have been listed and indexed by both their **Generic** and **Trade (Brand)** names for easy accessibility.

In addition to adverse drug reactions, there are many severe, hazardous **interactions** between two or more drugs. I have incorporated only the clinically important, potentially hazardous drug interactions that can trigger potential harm, and could be life-threatening. These interactions are predictable and well documented in controlled studies; they should be avoided.

For each drug, I have listed the known adverse side effects – in the form of drug reactions – that can develop from the use of the corresponding drug. These include reactions involving the skin, hair, nails, eyes, hematopoietic, cardiologic and other side effects. The section entitled 'other' includes such reactions as tinnitus, serotonin syndrome, depression, rhabdomyolysis, insomnia, and death.

The first part of the book lists, in alphabetical order, the **Generic** and **Trade** name drugs with their corresponding names for easy access to the **A-Z** section – the main body of the book. Next comes a listing of the various **Classes** of drugs, and those **Generic** drugs that belong to each class. The last part of the book includes listings of common neurological reactions caused mainly by non-neurological drugs.

The major portion of the pocketbook – the body of the work – lists the Generic drugs, herbals and supplements in alphabetical order and the adverse reactions that can arise from their use. The numbers in square brackets refer to the number of references recorded for each reaction. These references are available on my website (www.drugeruptiondata.com) or in the latest edition of the Drug Eruption Reference Manual.

USAGE, STYLE & CONVENTIONS EMPLOYED IN THIS POCKETBOOK

The **Generic Drug** name is at the top of each page.

The **Trade (Brand) Name(s)** are then listed alphabetically. When there are many **Trade Names**, the ten (or so) most commonly recognized ones are listed. This compilation lists and cross-references both the **Trade** *and* **Generic** names of all the cataloged drugs. Following the more common **Trade Name** drugs are recorded – in parentheses – the latest name of the pharmaceutical company that is marketing the drug.

Beneath the **Trade Name** listing is a list of Other **Common Trade Names**, those drugs from other countries. Then appear the **Indication(s)**, the **Category** in which the drug belongs, and the **Half-Life** of each drug, when known, and the **Potentially hazardous interactions** between drugs. On occasion, an important or pertinent **Note** will follow.

Reactions: These are the **Adverse Reactions** to the particular **Generic** drug.

They are classified into **Categories: Skin, Hair, Nails, Hematopoietic, Eyes, Cardiologic**, and **Other**. (**Other** refers to **Mucous Membrane, Teeth, Muscle** and various other **Reactions**.) **Reactions** are listed alphabetically under each heading. Alongside each **Reaction Pattern** are square bracketed numbers that refer to the number of references in the main Drug Eruption Reference Manual and my website. Numbers in round brackets refer to the incidence of the reaction, e.g. (3 cases) or (15%).

In the case of **herbals** and **supplements**, the format is slightly different. The herbals feature the scientific species and genus, purported indications and other uses, and interactions. Then follows the same format as the generic drugs.

There are occasions when there are very few adverse reactions to a specific drug. These drugs are still included, since there is often **positive significance in negative findings**.

Jerome Z. Litt, M.D.
May, 2005

INDEX OF GENERIC AND TRADE NAMES

Generic drug names are in **bold**

CLASSES OF DRUGS

Anticholinergics
biperiden
buclizine
clidinium
dicyclomine
glycopyrrolate
hyoscyamine
ipratropium
methantheline
procyclidine
propantheline
scopolamine
tiotropium
tolterodine
trihexyphenidyl

Anticonvulsants
acetazolamide
amobarbital
carbamazepine
clonazepam
ethosuximide
ethotoin
fosphenytoin
gabapentin
lamotrigine
levetiracetam
lorazepam
mephenytoin
mephobarbital
methsuximide
oxazepam
oxcarbazepine
paramethadione
pentobarbital
phensuximide
phenytoin
primidone
thiopental
tiagabine

topiramate
trimethadione
valproic acid
vigabatrin
zonisamide

Antimigraine
amitriptyline
frovatriptan
naratriptan
nicardipine
nifedipine
rizatriptan
sumatriptan
zolmitriptan

Anti-Parkinsonian
amantadine
apomorphine
benztropine
biperiden
bromocriptine
entacapone
levodopa
pergolide
pramipexole
procyclidine
ropinirole
selegiline
tolcapone
trihexyphenidyl

Neuromuscular blockers
atracurium
botulinum toxin (A & B)
cisatracurium
doxacurium
edrophonium
vecuronium

ACETAMINOPHEN

Synonyms: APAP; paracetamol
Trade names: Anacin-3 (Wyeth); Bromo-Seltzer; Darvocet-N (aaiPharma); Datril; Excedrin (Bristol-Myers Squibb); Liquiprin; Lorcet (Forest); Mapap; Neopap; Panadol (GSK); Percocet (Endo); Percogesic; Phenaphen; Sinutab; Tylenol (Ortho-McNeil); Valadol; Vicodin (Abbott)
Other common trade names: *Abenol; Anaflon; Ben-U-Ron; Doliprane; Geluprane; Panadol*
Indications: Pain, fever
Category: Non-narcotic antipyretic analgesic
Half-life: 1–3 hours
Clinically important, potentially hazardous interactions with: alcohol, cholestyramine, didanosine, dong quai, melatonin

Note: Acetaminophen is the active metabolite of phenacetin

Reactions

Skin
  Acute generalized exanthematous
    pustulosis (AGEP) [6]
  Angioedema (<1%) [6]
  Dermatitis [3]
  Diaphoresis
  Erythema [1]
  Erythema multiforme [2]
  Erythema nodosum (<1%)
  Exanthems [5]
  Exfoliative dermatitis [1]
  Fixed eruption (<1%) [29]
  Linear IgA dermatosis [1]
  Neutrophilic eccrine hidradenitis [1]
  Pemphigus [1]
  Penile edema [1]
  Photosensitivity [1]
  Pigmented purpuric eruption (Schamberg's
    disease) [1]
  Pityriasis rosea [1]
  Pruritus [2]
  Purpura [6]
  Purpura fulminans [1]

  Rash (sic) (<1%)
  Sensitivity (sic) [1]
  Stevens–Johnson syndrome [2]
  Toxic epidermal necrolysis [5]
  Urticaria [10]
  Vasculitis [2]

Hair
  Hair – alopecia [1]

Nails
  Nails – changes (sic) [1]

Hematopoietic
  Hemophilia [1]

Cardiovascular
  Flushing [1]

Other
  Anaphylactoid reactions [13]
  Death [2]
  Dysgeusia [1]
  Headache
  Hypersensitivity (<1%) [5]
  Rhabdomyolysis [3]

ACETAZOLAMIDE

Trade name: Diamox (Wyeth)
Other common trade names: *Acetazolam; Ak-Zol; Dazamide; Defiltran; Diuramid; Novo-Zolamide*
Indications: Epilepsy, glaucoma
Category: Anticonvulsant; Carbonic anhydrase inhibitor; Sulfonamide diuretic
Half-life: 2–6 hours
Clinically important, potentially hazardous interactions with: ephedra, lithium

---

Reactions

Skin
  Acute generalized exanthematous
    pustulosis (AGEP) [2]
  Bullous eruption (<1%) [1]
  Erythema multiforme [2]
  Exanthems [2]
  Frostbite [1]
  Lupus erythematosus [1]
  Photosensitivity
  Pruritus
  Purpura [1]
  Pustular psoriasis [1]
  Pustules [1]
  Rash (sic) (<1%)
  Rosacea [1]
  Stevens–Johnson syndrome
  Toxic epidermal necrolysis (<1%) [1]

Urticaria

Hair
  Hair – hirsutism [1]

Hematopoietic
  Thrombocytopenia [1]

Other
  Ageusia
  Anaphylactoid reactions [3]
  Anosmia
  Dysgeusia (>10%) (metallic taste) [3]
  Extravasation [1]
  Headache
  Myalgia [1]
  Paresthesias (<1%) [1]
  Tinnitus
  Xerostomia (<1%)

*Note: Acetazolamide is a sulfonamide and can be absorbed systemically. Sulfonamides can produce severe, possibly fatal, reactions such as toxic epidermal necrolysis and Stevens–Johnson syndrome

ADALIMUMAB

Synonym: D2E7
Trade name: Humira (Abbott)
Indications: Rheumatoid arthritis
Category: Anti-TNF-alpha monoclonal antibody
Half-life: 10–20 days

Reactions

Skin
  Allergic reactions (sic) (1%)

Carcinoma
Cellulitis

Erysipelas
Erythema multiforme [1]
Flu-like syndrome (7%)
Fungal dermatitis
Herpes zoster
Infections (5%)
Lupus erythematosus (<0.1%)
Lymphoma [1]
Melanoma
Peripheral edema
Rash (sic) (12%)
Upper respiratory infection (17%)

Other
Back pain (6%) [1]
Death
Headache
Injection-site edema (15.2%)
Injection-site erythema (15.2%)
Injection-site pain (12%)
Myasthenia
Paresthesias
Tendinitis
Tremor
Tuberculosis [1]

Note: TNF blocking agents may lead to serious infections, lymphoma, or fatalities, particularly in patients receiving concomitant immunosuppressive therapy. Patients should be evaluated for latent tuberculosis prior to treatment with adalimumab.

ALENDRONATE

Trade name: Fosamax (Merck)
Other common trade name: *Fosalan*
Indications: Osteoporosis in postmenopausal women, Paget's disease
Category: Biphosphonate; Inhibitor of bone resorption
Half-life: >10 years

Reactions

Skin
Erythema (<1%) [1]
Erythema gyratum [1]
Erythema multiforme [1]
Exanthems [1]
Fixed eruption [1]
Peripheral edema
Petechiae [1]
Pruritus (0.6%) [2]
Rash (sic) (<1%) [5]

Eyes
Conjunctivitis [1]
Ocular inflammation [1]

Ocular stinging [1]
Uveitis [1]
Visual disturbances [1]

Other
Abdominal pain [1]
Dysgeusia (0.6%) [1]
Hallucinations [1]
Headache
Hypersensitivity [1]
Oral ulceration [2]
Seizures [1]

ALFENTANIL

Trade name: Alfenta (Akorn)
Other common trade name: *Rapifen*
Indications: General anesthesia, post-operative pain
Category: Narcotic agonist analgesic
Half-life: 83–97 minutes (adults)
Clinically important, potentially hazardous interactions with: erythromycin, ranitidine, ritonavir

---

Reactions

Skin
  Clammy skin (<1%)
  Pruritus (<1%) [1]
  Rash (sic) (<1%)
  Shivering (3–9%) [1]
  Urticaria (<1%)

Cardiovascular
  Bradycardia [2]
  Hypotension [1]

Other
  Dysesthesia

ALMOTRIPTAN

Trade name: Axert (Ortho-McNeil)
Indications: Migraine headaches
Category: Serotonin 5-Ht1d receptor agonist
Half-life: 3–4 hours
Clinically important, potentially hazardous interactions with: dihydroergotamine, ergotamine, ketoconazole, methysergide

---

Reactions

Skin
  Chills (<1%)
  Dermatitis
  Diaphoresis (<1%)
  Erythema (<1%)
  Flu-like syndrome (12%) [1]
  Photosensitivity (<1%)
  Pruritus (<1%)
  Rash (sic) (<1%)
  Upper respiratory infection (20%)

Other
  Arthralgia (<1%)
  Bone or joint pain [1]
  Depression (<1%)
  Dizziness [1]
  Dysgeusia (<1%)
  Fatigue [1]
  Headache
  Hyperesthesia (<1%)
  Injection-site irritation [1]
  Myalgia (<1%)
  Paresthesias (1%) [3]
  Parosmia (<1%)
  Sialorrhea (<1%)
  Tinnitus (<1%)
  Xerostomia (1%) [1]

ALTEPLASE

Trade name: Activase (Genentech)
Other common trade names: *Actilyse; Activocin; Lysatec-rt-PA*
Indications: Acute myocardial infarction, acute pulmonary embolism
Category: Thrombolytic (tissue plasminogen activator)
Half-life: 30–45 minutes
Clinically important, potentially hazardous interactions with: nitroglycerin, ticlopidine

Reactions

Skin
  Angioedema [4]
  Purpura (<1%) [1]
  Rash (sic) (<0.02%)
  Urticaria (<1%) [1]

Hematopoietic
  Ecchymoses (1–10%)

Other
  Anaphylactoid reactions (<0.02%) [3]
  Death [1]
  Gingivitis (<1%)
  Headache
  Hypersensitivity [1]

ALTRETAMINE

Synonym: hexamethylmelamine
Trade name: Hexalen (MGI)
Other common trade names: *Hexamethylmelamin; Hexastat; Hexinawas*
Indications: Palliative treatment of recurrent ovarian cancer
Category: Antineoplastic
Half-life: 13 hours
Clinically important, potentially hazardous interactions with: aldesleukin

Reactions

Skin
  Dermatitis
  Exanthems
  Pruritus (<1%)
  Rash (sic) (<1%)

Hair
  Hair – alopecia (<1%)

Other
  Mucocutaneous reactions (sic) [1]
  Paresthesias [1]
  Tremor (<1%)

AMANTADINE

Trade name: Symmetrel (Endo)
Other common trade names: *Amixx; Endantadine; Grippin-Merz; Mantadix; PK-Merz; Protexin; Tregor*
Indications: Parkinsonism, influenza A viral infection
Category: Antidyskinetic; Antiparkinsonian; Antiviral
Half-life: 10–28 hours
Clinically important, potentially hazardous interactions with: memantine

Note: Fifty to 90% of patients receiving amantadine for Parkinsonism develop 'a more or less livedo reticularis'

Reactions

Skin
  Dermatitis (0.1%) [20]
  Discoloration [1]
  Eczema [1]
  Edema [1]
  Erythema multiforme [1]
  Exanthems [1]
  Livedo reticularis (50–90%) [15]
  Peripheral edema [5]
  Photosensitivity [2]
  Pruritus (<1%) [2]
  Rash (sic) (<1%)
  Urticaria

Hair
  Hair – alopecia [1]
  Hair – hypertrichosis [1]

Nails
  Nails – growth [1]

Eyes
  Eyelid edema

Cardiovascular
  QT prolongation [1]

Other
  Headache
  Xerostomia (1–10%) [3]

AMITRIPTYLINE

Trade names: Elavil (AstraZeneca); Limbitrol (Valeant)
Other common trade names: *Amineurin; Domical; Laroxyl; Lentizol; Levate; Novotriptyn; Saroten; Tryptanol; Tryptizol*
Indications: Depression
Category: Antimigraine; Tricyclic antidepressant
Half-life: 10–25 hours
Clinically important, potentially hazardous interactions with: amprenavir, clonidine, ephedra, epinephrine, eucalyptus, guanethidine, isocarboxazid, linezolid, MAO inhibitors, phenelzine, quinolones, sparfloxacin, st john's wort, tranylcypromine

Limbitrol is amitriptyline and chlordiazepoxide

Reactions

Skin
  Acne
  Allergic reactions (sic) (<1%)
  Angioedema [1]
  Bullous eruption (<1%) [1]
  Dermatitis [1]
  Dermatitis herpetiformis [1]
  Diaphoresis (1–10%) [1]
  Edema [1]
  Erythema
  Erythema annulare centrifugum [1]
  Erythroderma [1]
  Exanthems
  Exfoliative dermatitis
  Facial edema
  Fixed eruption [1]
  Lichen planus [1]
  Lupus erythematosus [1]
  Necrosis [1]
  Petechiae
  Photosensitivity (<1%) [3]
  Pigmentation [3]
  Pruritus [3]
  Purpura [2]
  Rash (sic)
  Urticaria
  Vasculitis [1]

Hair
  Hair – alopecia (<1%) [1]

Eyes
  Nystagmus [1]

Cardiovascular
  Congestive heart failure [1]
  Flushing
  QT prolongation [1]
  Torsades de pointes [1]

Other
  Ageusia
  Anaphylactoid reactions
  Black tongue
  Bromhidrosis
  Depression [1]
  Dysgeusia (>10%)
  Galactorrhea (<1%)
  Glossitis
  Gynecomastia (<1%)
  Headache
  Hypersensitivity [1]
  Lymphoid hyperplasia [1]
  Oral mucosal eruption [1]
  Paresthesias
  Parkinsonism
  Pseudolymphoma [2]
  Rhabdomyolysis [1]
  Seizures [1]
  Sialopenia [1]
  Sialorrhea
  Stomatitis [1]
  Stomatopyrosis
  Tardive dyskinesia [1]
  Tinnitus
  Tongue edema
  Tremor
  Vaginitis
  Xerostomia (>10%) [4]

AMOBARBITAL

Trade name: Amytal
Other common trade names: *Amytal Sodium; Isoamitil Sedante; Neur-Amyl; Novambarb; Sodium Amytal*
Indications: Insomnia, sedation
Category: Anticonvulsant; Barbiturate sedative-hypnotic
Half-life: initial: 40 minutes; terminal: 20 hours
Clinically important, potentially hazardous interactions with: alcohol, dicumarol, ethanolamine, warfarin

---

Reactions

Skin
  Acne
  Angioedema
  Bullous eruption
  Erythema [1]
  Exanthems
  Exfoliative dermatitis (<1%)
  Photosensitivity
  Purpura
  Rash (sic) (<1%)
  Stevens–Johnson syndrome (<1%)

  Toxic epidermal necrolysis [1]
  Urticaria (<1%)

Other
  Headache
  Hypersensitivity
  Injection-site pain (>10%)
  Rhabdomyolysis [1]
  Serum sickness
  Thrombophlebitis (<1%)

AMYL NITRITE

Synonym: isoamyl nitrite
Trade name: Amyl Nitrite
Other common trade name: *Nitrit*
Indications: Angina pectoris
Category: Antianginal; Coronary vasodilator
Half-life: N/A
Clinically important, potentially hazardous interactions with: furosemide, sildenafil

---

Reactions

Skin
  Allergic reactions (sic) [1]
  Dermatitis [3]
  Diaphoresis
  Edema
  Pallor
  Rash (sic) (<1%)

Cardiovascular
  Flushing (1–10%)

Other
  Headache

ANAKINRA

Synonym: IL-1RA
Trade name: Kineret (Amgen)
Indications: Rheumatoid arthritis
Category: Disease modifying antirheumatic (DMARD); Interleukin-1 receptor antagonist
Half-life: 4–6 hours
Clinically important, potentially hazardous interactions with: etanercept

Reactions

Skin
Flu-like syndrome (6%)
Infections (40%) [2]
Upper respiratory infection (4%)

Hematopoietic
Injection-site ecchymoses

Other
Headache

Hypersensitivity
Injection-site erythema
Injection-site inflammation
Injection-site pain
Injection-site reactions (sic) (71%) [8]
Sinusitis (7%)

APOMORPHINE

Trade names: Apokyn (Mylan Bertek); Uprima (Abbott)
Indications: Parkinsonism, Erectile dysfunction
Category: Antiparkinsonian; Non-ergot dopamine receptor agonist
Half-life: 40 minutes
Clinically important, potentially hazardous interactions with: alcohol, antihypertensives, vasodilators

Reactions

Skin
Dermatitis [1]
Diaphoresis (>5%)
Nodular eruption [1]
Peripheral edema (10%)
Pigmentation [1]

Hematopoietic
Ecchymoses (>5%)

Cardiovascular
Atrial fibrillation [1]
Chest pain (15%)
Congestive heart failure (>5%)

Other
Anxiety (>5%)
Arthralgia (>5%)
Back pain (>5%)
Depression (>5%)
Diaphoresis [1]
Dizziness (20%) [2]
Dysgeusia [1]
Dyskinesia (35%) [3]
Fatigue (>5%)
Hallucinations (10%) [2]
Headache (>5%) [2]
Injection-site reactions (sic) [2]

Limb pain (>5%)
Panniculitis [2]
Pneumonia (>5%)
Priapism [1]

Rhinorrhea (20%)
Urinary tract infection (>5%)
Yawning (40%) [2]

Note: Apomorphine contains sodium metabisulfite which is capable of causing anaphylactoid reactions in patients with sulfite allergy

ASPIRIN

Synonyms: acetylsalicylic acid; ASA

Trade names: Aggrenox (Boehringer Ingelheim); Alka-Seltzer; Anacin (Wyeth); Ascriptin (Novartis) (Wallace); Aspergum; Coricidin D; Darvon Compound (aaiPharma); Ecotrin (GSK); Empirin; Equagesic (Women First); Excedrin (Bristol-Myers Squibb); Fiorinal (Watson); Gelprin; Halfprin; Measurin; Norgesic (3M); Robaxisal; Soma Compound (MedPointe); Talwin Compound (Sanofi-Aventis); Vanquish

Other common trade names: ASA; Aspro; ASS; Bex; *Caprin; Claragine; Disprin; Ecotrin; Novasen; Rhonal*

Indications: Pain, fever, inflammation

Category: Nonsteroidal anti-inflammatory (NSAID) analgesic; Salicylate

Half-life: 15–20 minutes

Clinically important, potentially hazardous interactions with: anticoagulants, bismuth, boswellia, capsicum, cholestyramine, devil's claw, dicumarol, etodolac, **evening primrose,** ginkgo biloba, ginseng, heparin, ibuprofen, indomethacin, ketoprofen, ketorolac, methotrexate, NSAIDs, **phellodendron, resveratrol,** reteplase, sermorelin, **sulfites,** tirofiban, urokinase, valdecoxib, valproic acid, verapamil, warfarin

Aggrenox is aspirin and dipyridamole

Reactions

Skin

Acute generalized exanthematous pustulosis (AGEP) [1]
Allergic reactions (sic) (<1%) (with dipyridamole) [1]
Angioedema (1–5%) [21]
Baboon syndrome [1]
Bullous eruption (<1%) [4]
Dermatitis herpetiformis [1]
Dermatomyositis [1]
Diaphoresis
Erythema multiforme (<1%) [9]
Erythema nodosum (<1%) [9]
Erythroderma [1]

Exanthems [11]
Exfoliative dermatitis [1]
Fixed eruption (<1%) [21]
Genital herpes [1]
Graft-versus-host reaction [1]
Granulomas [1]
Herpes simplex [1]
Lichenoid eruption [2]
Parapsoriasis [1]
Pemphigus [1]
Petechiae [1]
Photo-recall [1]
Pigmented purpuric eruption [1]
Pityriasis rosea [2]

Pruritus [6]
Psoriasis [2]
Purpura [7]
Pustular psoriasis [2]
Rash (sic) (1–10%)
Stevens–Johnson syndrome [4]
Toxic epidermal necrolysis (<1%) [9]
Ulcerations (<1%) (with dipyridamole)
Urticaria (1–10%) [62]
Vasculitis [3]

Hair
Hair – alopecia [1]

Eyes
Ocular hemorrhage [1]
Periorbital edema [3]

Cardiovascular
Flushing [1]

Other
Ageusia (<1%) (with dipyridamole)
Anaphylactoid reactions (1–10%) [6]
Aphthous stomatitis [3]
Dysgeusia
Gingivitis (<1%) (with dipyridamole)
Headache
Hypersensitivity [3]
Myalgia (1.2%) (with dipyridamole)
Oral burn [1]
Oral lichen planus [1]
Oral mucosal eruption [3]
Oral ulceration [4]
Paresthesias (<1%) (with dipyridamole)
Pseudolymphoma [1]
Pseudoporphyria [1]
Tinnitus

ATENOLOL

Trade names: Tenoretic (AstraZeneca); Tenormin (AstraZeneca)
Other common trade names: *Antipressan; Apo-Atenol; AteHexal; Atendol; Evitocor; Noten; Novo-Atenol; Nu-Atenol; Taro-Atenol; Tenolin; Tenormine*
Indications: Angina, hypertension, acute myocardial infarction
Category: Antianginal; Antihypertensive; Beta-adrenoceptor blocker
Half-life: 6–7 hours (adults)
Clinically important, potentially hazardous interactions with: alfuzosin, clonidine, epinephrine, verapamil

Tenoretic is atenolol and chlorthalidone

Reactions

Skin
Acrocyanosis [1]
Dermatitis [1]
Diaphoresis
Edema
Erythema multiforme
Exanthems
Facial edema
Fixed eruption [1]
Grinspan's syndrome* [1]
Hyperkeratosis (palms and soles)

Lichenoid eruption [1]
Lupus erythematosus [2]
Necrosis [3]
Papulo-nodular lesions [1]
Photosensitivity
Pityriasis rubra pilaris [1]
Pruritus (1–5%)
Psoriasis [7]
Purpura
Pustular psoriasis [1]
Rash (sic) [1]

Raynaud's phenomenon [1]
Toxic epidermal necrolysis
Urticaria [2]
Vasculitis [1]
Vitiligo
Xerosis

Hair
Hair – alopecia [1]

Nails
Nails – dystrophy
Nails – onycholysis
Nails – pigmentation
Nails – splinter hemorrhages [1]

Eyes
Oculo-mucocutaneous syndrome [1]

Cardiovascular
Arrhythmias [1]
Atrial fibrillation [1]
Bradycardia [5]
Hypotension [1]
Stroke [1]

Other
Anaphylactoid reactions [1]
Death [1]
Oral lichenoid eruption [1]
Peyronie's disease
Pseudolymphoma [1]

*Note: Grinspan's syndrome: the triad of oral lichen planus, diabetes mellitus, and hypertension

ATRACURIUM

Trade name: Tracrium (Abbott)
Indications: Neuromuscular blockade, endotracheal intubation
Category: Neuromuscular blocker; Skeletal muscle relaxant
Half-life: initial: 2 minutes; terminal: 20 minutes
Clinically important, potentially hazardous interactions with: amikacin, aminoglycosides, anesthetics, antibiotics, gentamicin, halothane, kanamycin, neomycin, piperacillin, streptomycin, tobramycin

Reactions

Skin
Allergic reactions (sic) [2]
Edema
Erythema (<1%)
Pruritus (<1%)
Urticaria (<1%)

Cardiovascular
Flushing (1–10%)

Other
Injection-site reactions (sic)

ATROPINE SULFATE

Trade names: Belladenal; Bellergal-S; Butibel; Donnagel; Donnatal; Donnazyme; Isopto Atropine; Lofene; Logen; Lomanate; Lomotil (Pfizer); Urised
Other common trade names: *Atropine Martinet; Atropt; Chibro-Atropine; Isopto; Tropyn Z; Vitatropine*
Indications: Salivation, sinus bradycardia, uveitis, peptic ulcer
Category: Anticholinesterase
Half-life: 2–3 hours
Clinically important, potentially hazardous interactions with: anticholinergics

---

Reactions

Skin
  Adverse effects (sic) [1]
  Allergic reactions (sic) [2]
  Bullous eruption [1]
  Dermatitis [3]
  Eccrine hidrocystomas [1]
  Erythema (sheet-like)
  Erythema multiforme (<1%) [2]
  Exanthems
  Exfoliative dermatitis [1]
  Fixed eruption [2]
  Hypohidrosis (>10%) [1]
  Photosensitivity (1–10%)
  Pruritus
  Rash (sic) (<1%)
  Stevens–Johnson syndrome [1]
  Urticaria [1]
  Xerosis

Eyes
  Eyelid edema

  Ocular allergic reactions (sic) [1]
  Periocular dermatitis [3]

Cardiovascular
  Arrhythmias [1]
  Atrial fibrillation [2]
  Bradycardia [2]
  Flushing [1]
  Myocardial ischemia [1]
  Tachycardia [3]
  Ventricular tachycardia [1]

Other
  Anaphylactoid reactions [1]
  Dry mucous membranes [1]
  Dysgeusia
  Headache
  Injection-site irritation (>10%)
  Tremor
  Xerostomia (>10%)

*Note: Many of the above trade name drugs contain phenobarbital, scopolamine, hyoscyamine, hydrocodone, methenamine, etc

AURANOFIN (See GOLD and GOLD COMPOUNDS)

AUROTHIOGLUCOSE (See GOLD and GOLD COMPOUNDS)

AZATHIOPRINE

Trade name: Imuran (Prometheus)
Other common trade names: Azamedac; Azamune; Azatrilem; Imuprin; Imurek; Imurel; Thioprine
Indications: Lupus nephritis, psoriatic arthritis, rheumatoid arthritis, autoimmune diseases, kidney transplant patients
Category: Immunosuppressant
Half-life: 12 minutes
Clinically important, potentially hazardous interactions with: allopurinol, chlorambucil, cyclophosphamide, cyclosporine, mycophenolate, olsalazine, vaccines, warfarin

---

Reactions

Skin
  Acanthosis nigricans [2]
  Acne [1]
  Allergic reactions (sic) [1]
  Angioedema [1]
  Basal cell carcinoma [1]
  Carcinoma [1]
  Chills (>10%)
  Dermatitis [3]
  Erythema [1]
  Erythema gyratum repens [2]
  Erythema multiforme [2]
  Erythema nodosum [2]
  Exanthems [10]
  Exfoliative dermatitis [1]
  Fixed eruption [1]
  Flu-like syndrome [1]
  Formication [1]
  Fungal dermatitis [1]
  Herpes simplex [3]
  Herpes zoster [7]
  Infections [4]
  Intraepidermal carcinoma [1]
  Kaposi's sarcoma [11]
  Keratoacanthoma [1]
  Lichenoid eruption [1]
  Neoplasms [1]
  Pemphigus foliaceus [1]
  Peripheral edema [1]
  Photosensitivity
  Pigmentation (sun-exposed skin) [1]
  Porokeratosis [4]
  Purpura
  Pyoderma gangrenosum [1]
  Rash (sic) (1–10%) [5]
  Raynaud's phenomenon
  Sarcoma [1]
  Scabies [4]
  Scleroderma [1]
  Squamous cell carcinoma [9]
  Stevens–Johnson syndrome [1]
  Tinea [3]
  Toxic epidermal necrolysis [1]
  Urticaria [5]
  Vasculitis [4]
  Viral infections [2]
  Warts [2]

Hair
  Hair – alopecia (<1%) [3]
  Hair – curly [1]

Nails
  Nails – discoloration (red lunulae) [1]
  Nails – onychomycosis [2]

Cardiovascular
  Atrial fibrillation [1]

Other
  Anaphylactoid reactions [1]
  Aphthous stomatitis (<1%)
  Cicatricial pemphigoid [1]
  Hypersensitivity (<1%)* [16]
  Lymphoproliferative disease [3]
  Myalgia (<1%)

Non-Hodgkin's lymphoma [1]
Oral ulceration [1]
Pneumonia [1]
Rhabdomyolysis [1]
Rheumatoid nodules [1]

Serum sickness
Stomatitis [1]
Tumors [8]
Xerostomia

BACLOFEN

Trade names: Baclofen (Watson); Lioresal (Medtronic)
Other common trade names: *Alpha-Baclofen; Baclon; Baclosal; Baklofen; Clofen; Dom-Baclofen; Gen-Baclofen; Lebic; Nu-Baclo; Pacifen; PMS-Baclofen; Spinax*
Indications: Spasticity resulting from multiple sclerosis
Category: Antispastic; Skeletal muscle relaxant
Half-life: 2.5–4 hours

Reactions

Skin
　Dermatitis
　Diaphoresis
　Exanthems [1]
　Facial edema
　Peripheral edema [1]
　Pruritus
　Rash (sic) (1–10%)
　Side effects (sic) (1–2%) [1]
　Urticaria [1]

Cardiovascular
　Flushing

Other
　Dysgeusia (<1%) [1]
　Headache
　Paresthesias (<1%)
　Tinnitus
　Xerostomia (<1%)

BALSALAZIDE

Trade name: Colazal (Salix)
Indications: Mild to moderately active ulcerative colitis
Category: Aminosalicylate anti-inflammatory
Half-life: N/A

Reactions

Skin
　Flu-like syndrome (1%)
　Pruritus
　Rash (sic)

Hair
　Hair – alopecia

Other
　Arthralgia (4%)
　Headache
　Hypersensitivity [1]
　Myalgia (1%)
　Xerostomia (1%)

BENZTROPINE

Trade name: Cogentin (Merck)
Other common trade names: *Akitan; Apo-Benzthioprine; Cogentine; Cogentinol; Phatropine; PMS-Benztropine*
Indications: Parkinsonism
Category: Antidyskinetic; Antiparkinsonian
Half-life: 6–48 hours
Clinically important, potentially hazardous interactions with: anticholinergics

Reactions

Skin
Exanthems
Hypohidrosis (>10%)
Photosensitivity (1–10%)
Pruritus
Rash (sic) (<1%)
Urticaria
Xerosis (>10%)

Other
Black tongue [1]
Death [1]
Dysgeusia [1]
Glossodynia
Paresthesias
Stomatodynia
Tinnitus
Xerostomia (>10%) [2]

BEPRIDIL

Trade name: Vascor (Ortho-McNeil)
Other common trade names: *Bapadin; Bepricol; Cordium; Cruor*
Indications: Angina pectoris
Category: Antianginal; Calcium channel blocker
Half-life: 24 hours
Clinically important, potentially hazardous interactions with: amprenavir, atazanavir, ciprofloxacin, enoxacin, epirubicin, fosamprenavir, gatifloxacin, lomefloxacin, **mistletoe**, moxifloxacin, norfloxacin, ofloxacin, quinolones, ritonavir, sparfloxacin

Reactions

Skin
Diaphoresis (<2%)
Edema (1–10%)
Irritation (sic)
Peripheral edema (<1%)
Rash (sic) (<2%) [1]

Cardiovascular
Tachycardia [1]
Torsades de pointes [1]

Other
Dysgeusia (<1%)
Myalgia (<1%)
Paresthesias (2.5%)
Tinnitus
Tremor (<9%)
Xerostomia (1–10%) [2]

BERGAMOT*

Scientific name: *Citrus aurantium ssp bergamia*
Family: Rutaceae
Trade and other common names: Bergamottin; Earl Grey tea; Florida Water; Kananga Water;
Neroli oil; Oil of bergamot
Category: Mild stimulant
Purported indications and other uses: Headache, bronchitis, vitiligo, mycosis fungoides,
psoriasis (in conjunction with UVA), insecticide, essential oil in perfumery, cosmetics, flavoring
Half-life: N/A

*Note: two distinct species are known by the common name of bergamot. This profile does not
refer to *Monarda didyma*

Reactions

Skin
  Adverse effects (sic) [1]
  Berloque dermatitis [2]
  Bullous eruption [1]
  Burning [1]
  Dermatitis [2]

Erythema [1]
Photosensitivity [3]
Phototoxicity [7]
Pigmentation [1]
Tumors [1]
Vesiculation [1]

Note: Oil of bergamot possesses photosensitive and melanogenic properties because of the
presence of furocoumarins, primarily bergapten (5-methoxypsoralen [5-MOP]). Its use is
restricted or banned in many countries

BIPERIDEN

Trade name: Akineton (Par)
Other common trade names: *Biperen; Bipiden; Dekinet; Desiperiden; Dyskinon*
Indications: Parkinsonism
Category: Anticholinergic; Antiparkinsonian
Half-life: 18–24 hours
Clinically important, potentially hazardous interactions with: anticholinergics

Reactions

Skin
  Dermatitis [1]
  Diaphoresis [1]
  Exanthems
  Rash (sic)
  Urticaria

Cardiovascular
  Flushing

Other
  Glossodynia
  Paresthesias
  Stomatodynia
  Xerostomia

BISOPROLOL

Trade names: Zebeta (Barr); Ziac (Barr)
Other common trade names: *Concor; Cordalin; Detensiel; Emcor; Fondril; Monocor; Soprol*
Indications: Hypertension
Category: Beta-adrenoceptor blocker
Half-life: 9–12 hours

Ziac is bisoprolol and hydrochlorothiazide

Reactions

Skin
  Acne
  Angioedema
  Diaphoresis (1%)
  Eczema
  Edema (3%)
  Exanthems
  Exfoliative dermatitis
  Facial edema
  Lupus erythematosus
  Peripheral edema (1–10%)
  Photosensitivity
  Pigmentation
  Pruritus
  Psoriasis
  Purpura
  Rash (sic) (1–10%)
  Raynaud's phenomenon (1–10%)
  Urticaria
  Xerosis

Hair
  Hair – alopecia

Nails
  Nails – pigmentation

Cardiovascular
  Flushing

Other
  Anaphylactoid reactions
  Dysgeusia
  Headache
  Hyperesthesia (1.5%)
  Myalgia (1–10%)
  Paresthesias
  Peyronie's disease
  Tinnitus
  Xerostomia (1.3%)

BLACK COHOSH

Scientific names: *Actaea macrotys; Actaea racemosa; Cimicifuga racemosa*
Family: Ranunculaceae
Trade and other common names: Baneberry; Black Snake root; Bugbane; Bugwort; Macrotys; Rattletop; Rattleweed; Remifemin (PhytoPharmica/Enzymatic Therapy; Schaper & Brummer); Shengma; Squawroot
Category: Phytoestrogen
Purported indications and other uses: Anxiety, arthritis, asthma, cardiovascular and circulatory problems, climacteric, menstrual and premenstrual disorders, colds, cough, constipation, depression, kidney disorders, malaria, sore throat, tinnitus
Half-life: N/A
Clinically important, potentially hazardous interactions with: estrogens, salicylates, tamoxifen

Reactions

Skin
  Diaphoresis [2]
  Jaundice [1]
  Petechiae (forearms)
  Pruritus [1]
  Rash (sic) [1]

Other
  Arthralgia (overdose)
  Dizziness [1]
  Mastodynia [1]
  Seizures [3]
  Tremor (overdose)

Note: In 2001, the American College of Obstetricians and Gynecologists stated that black cohosh might be helpful in the short term (6 months or less) for women with vasomotor symptoms of menopause

BLOODROOT

Scientific name: *Sanguinaria canadensis*
Family: Papaveraceae
Trade and other common names: Coon Root; Indian Plant; Indian Red Paint; Red Puccoon; Red Root; Snakebite; Sweet Slumber; Tetterwort; Viadent
Category: Anti-inflammatory; Antispasmodic
Purported indications and other uses: Oral: emetic, cathartic, expectorant. Topical: debriding agent, bronchitis, asthma, croup, laryngitis, pharyngitis, scabies, eczema, athlete's foot, nasal polyps, rheumatism, fever, anemia
Half-life: N/A

Reactions

Skin
  Dermatitis [1]
  Irritation (sic)

Other
  Keratoses [1]
  Leukoplakia [2]

BLUE COHOSH

Scientific name: *Caulophyllum thalictroides*
Family: Berberidaceae
Trade and other common names: Beechdrops; Blue ginseng; Blueberry root; Papoose root;
Squawroot; Yellow ginseng
Category: Anthelmintic; Antispasmodic diuretic; Diaphoretic; Expectorant; Oxytocic
Purported indications and other uses: Rheumatism, dropsy, epilepsy, hysteria, uterine
inflammation, thrush, menopause, headache, sexual debility, aphthous stomatitis, laxative, colic,
sore throat, hiccups
Half-life: N/A
Clinically important, potentially hazardous interactions with: cardioactive drugs

Reactions

Skin
  Allergic reactions (sic)
  Diaphoresis [1]

Other
  Mucosal irritation
  Myalgia [1]
  Shock [1]

Note: Cohosh is from the Algonquin word 'rough', referring to the appearance of the roots. It is
a toxic herb and should not be confused with the safer, unrelated herb, Black Cohosh

BOTULINUM TOXIN (A & B)

Trade names: Botox (Allergan); Dysport (Ipsen); Myobloc (Solstice)
Indications: Blepharospasm, hemifacial spasm, spasmodic torticollis, sialorrhea, hyperhidrosis,
strabismus, oromandibular dystonia, cervical dystonia, spasmodic dysphonia. Cosmetic application
for wrinkles
Category: Neuromuscular blocker; Toxin
Half-life: 3–6 months

Reactions

Skin
  Acne
  Allergic reactions (sic)
  Depigmentation [1]
  Erythema multiforme
  Flu-like syndrome (2–10%) [4]
  Hematomas [2]
  Hypohidrosis [1]
  Infections (13–19%)
  Intertrigo [1]
  Peripheral edema (1–10%)

  Pruritus (1–10%)
  Psoriasis
  Purpura (1–10%)
  Rash (sic)
  Urticaria

Eyes
  Ectropion [1]
  Entropion
  Eyelid edema [1]
  Ptosis (14–20%) [3]
  Punctate keratitis [1]

Xerophthalmia (6.3%) [1]

Hematopoietic
Injection-site ecchymoses [2]

Other
Anaphylactoid reactions [1]
Arthralgia (<7%)
Death
Depression [1]
Dysgeusia (1–10%) [1]
Dysphagia [1]
Headache
Hyperesthesia (1–10%)
Injection-site bruising [2]

Injection-site burning [1]
Injection-site edema [3]
Injection-site pain (2–10%) [6]
Injection-site rash (sic) [1]
Limb pain
Neck pain [1]
Oral candidiasis [1]
Pain (6–13%) [3]
Stomatitis (1–10%)
Tinnitus (1–10%)
Tremor (1–10%) [1]
Vulvovaginal candidiasis (1–10%)
Xerostomia (3–34%) [4]

Note: An antitoxin is available in the event of overdose or misinjection

BROMOCRIPTINE

Trade name: Parlodel (Novartis)
Other common trade names: *Apo-Bromocriptine; Bromed; Cryocriptina; Kripton; Parilac; Pravidel; Serocryptin*
Indications: Amenorrhea, parkinsonism, infertility
Category: Antidyskinetic; Antihyperprolactinemic; Antiparkinsonian; Dopamine agonist; Growth hormone suppressant; Infertility therapy adjunct; Lactation inhibitor
Half-life: initial: 6–8 hours; terminal: 50 hours
Clinically important, potentially hazardous interactions with: erythromycin, pseudoephedrine, sympathomimetics

Reactions

Skin
Exanthems
Livedo reticularis [3]
Morphea [1]
Nodular eruption
Purpura
Rash (sic)
Raynaud's phenomenon (1–10%) [5]
Scleroderma [2]
Urticaria
Vasculitis [1]

Hair
Hair – alopecia [2]

Cardiovascular
Flushing [1]
Hypertension [1]

Other
Anaphylactoid reactions [1]
Dysgeusia (metallic taste)
Erythromelalgia [4]
Headache [1]
Paresthesias [1]
Priapism (clitoral)
Pseudolymphoma [1]
Seizures [2]
Stomatopyrosis [1]
Xerostomia (4–10%) [2]

BUCLIZINE

Trade names: Bucladin-S; Vibazine
Other common trade names: *Aphilan; Buclixin; Longifene; Odetin; Postafeno; Vibazina*
Indications: Motion sickness, nausea/vomiting
Category: Anticholinergic; Antiemetic; Antihistamine
Half-life: N/A
Clinically important, potentially hazardous interactions with: aprobarbital, butabarbital, chloral hydrate, ethchlorvynol, mephobarbital, pentobarbital, phenobarbital, phenothiazines, primidone, secobarbital, zolpidem

---
Reactions

Other
  Tremor

                  Xerostomia

BUTORPHANOL

Trade name: Stadol (Bristol-Myers Squibb)
Other common trade names: *Biforal; Busphen; Stadol NS*
Indications: Pain, migraine
Category: Analgesic; Narcotic
Half-life: 2.5–4 hours
Clinically important, potentially hazardous interactions with: cimetidine

---
Reactions

Skin
  Clammy skin
  Diaphoresis (1–10%)
  Edema (<1%)
  Exanthems
  Gooseflesh
  Pruritus (1–10%) [2]
  Rash (sic) (<1%)
  Urticaria (<1%)

Cardiovascular
  Flushing (1–10%)

Other
  Dysgeusia (3–9%)
  Headache
  Injection-site reactions (sic)
  Paresthesias
  Tinnitus
  Xerostomia (3–9%)

BUTTERBUR

Scientific names: *Petasites hybridus; Petasites officinalis*
Family: Asteraceae; Compositae
Trade and other common names: Blatterdock; bog rhubarb; bogshorn; butterdock; butterfly dock; capdockin; flapperdock; Petadolex* (Weber & Weber)
Category: Anodyne; Anti-inflammatory; Antispasmodic
Purported indications and other uses: Allergic rhinitis, asthma, bronchitis, chills, cough, dysmenorrhea, hay fever, headache, heart tonic, migraine, peptic ulcer, appetite stimulant, irritable bladder, poultice for wounds or skin ulcers
Half-life: N/A

*Note: Petadolex formulation has had the potentially carcinogenic pyrrolizidine alkaloids removed

Reactions

Skin
Edema (<0.1%) [2]
Erythema (<0.1%) [2]
Pruritus (<1%) [1]
Rash (sic) [2]

Eyes
Ocular pruritus (<1%) [1]

Other
Hypersensitivity (<0.1%) [2]

CABERGOLINE

Trade name: Dostinex (Pfizer)
Indications: Hyperprolactinemia, parkinsonism
Category: Dopamine receptor agonist; Ergot alkaloid
Half-life: 63–69 hours

Reactions

Skin
Acne (1%) [1]
Facial edema (1%)
Fixed eruption [1]
Flu-like syndrome (1%)
Peripheral edema (1%)
Pruritus (1%)

Hair
Hair – alopecia [1]

Eyes
Periorbital edema (1%)

Cardiovascular
Hot flashes (3%)

Other
Mastodynia (2%)
Paresthesias (5%)
Toothache (1%)
Xerostomia (2%)

CAFFEINE

Scientific names: *Coffea arabica; Coffea canephora; Coffea robusta; Cola acuminata; guarana (Paullinia cupana); Thea sinensis; Theobroma cacao*

Family: Rubiales

Trade and other common names: 1, 3, 7 trimethylxanthine; Anacin; Aqua-Ban; Black tea; Cafergot; Cola; Coryban-D; Darvon Compound; Dexatrim; Dristan; Elsinore; Endolor; Esgic; Excedrin; Fioricet; Fiorinal; Midol; Migralam; NoDoz; Norgesic; Norgesic Forte; Synalgos-DC; Synalgos-DC-A; Triaminicin; Vanquish; Vivarin (GSK). Ingredient in: Adipokinetix

Category: CNS stimulant; Somnolytic

Purported indications and other uses: with ergotamine for migraine, with NSAIDs in analgesics, headache, respiratory depression in neonates, postprandial hypotension, enhances seizure duration in electroconvulsive therapy. Ingredient in cough and cold remedies

Half-life: 2–7 hours

Clinically important, potentially hazardous interactions with: carbamazepine, cimetidine, clozapine, **ephedra**, fluorides, **ginseng, guarana,** idrocilamide, methoxsalen, mexiletine, phenylpropanolamine, zonisamide

Note: Caffeine is an addictive psychoactive substance. Spontaneous abortion and low birthweight babies have occurred in pregnant women consuming 150 mg caffeine per day. Abuse can lead to cardiac damage or death

Physical Dependence & Withdrawal of Caffeine

Common symptoms of caffeine withdrawal are headache; drowsiness; yawning, impaired concentration; lassitude; irritability; decreased contentedness, well-being and self-confidence; decreased sociability; flu-like symptoms; muscle aches and stiffness; hot or cold spells; nausea or vomiting; and blurred vision

---

Reactions

Skin
Angioedema
Bullous eruption
Burning (feet) [1]
Chills [1]
Exfoliative dermatitis
Facial edema
Pemphigus [1]
Pruritus
Purpura
Rash (sic)
Rosacea [1]
Urticaria [5]
Xanthoderma

Hematopoietic
Ecchymoses

Cardiovascular
Arrhythmias [1]
Atrial fibrillation [2]

Other
Anaphylactoid reactions [3]
Death (from abuse/overdose) [20]
Depression [2]
Hallucinations [1]
Headache
Hypersensitivity [1]
Paresthesias [1]
Rhabdomyolysis [5]
Seizures [1]
Tic disorder [1]
Tremor [4]
Xerostomia [1]

CAPSICUM

Scientific names: *Capsicum annuum; Capsicum baccatum; Capsicum chinense; Capsicum frutescens; Capsicum pubescens*

Family: Solanaceae

Trade and other common names: African chili; Bell pepper; Bird pepper; Capsaicin; Capsicool; Capsin; Capzasin-P; Cayenne; Cayenne Pepper; Chili; Dolorac; Goat's pod; Ici Fructus; Jalapeno; Louisiana long pepper; No Pain-HP; Oleoresin; Pain Doctor (with methyl-salicylate and menthol); Pain-X; Paprika; Pimento; R-Gel; Zanzibar pepper; Zostrix

Category: Antiseptic; Spasmolytic; Stimulant; Stomachic

Purported indications and other uses: nausea, neuropathic pain, osteoarthritis, fibromyalgia, anticarcinogen, rheumatoid arthritis, diabetic neuropathy, postherpetic neuralgia (shingles), psoriasis, pruritus, vitiligo, dyspepsia, flatulence, ulcers, stomach cramps, hypertension, improved circulation, weight-loss.

Half-life: N/A

Clinically important, potentially hazardous interactions with: ACE inhibitors, antiplatelet drugs, aspirin, disulfiram, heparin, latex, salicylic acid, theophylline, warfarin

Note: Pepper spray or gas contains 5% oleoresin capsicum (OC). It is used by police and in personal defense sprays

Reactions

Skin

Acute febrile neutrophilic dermatosis (Sweet's syndrome) [1]
Adverse effects (sic) [3]
Allergic reactions (sic) [3]
Bullous eruption [1]
Burning [4]
Dermatitis [3]
Diaphoresis [1]
Erosions [1]
Erythema [3]
Erythema multiforme [1]
Inflammation [1]
Irritation [1]
Pustules [1]
Sensitization [1]
Stinging [1]
Toxicoderma [1]
Urticaria [2]

Eyes

Conjunctivitis [3]
Lacrimation [1]
Ocular burning [1]
Rhinoconjunctivitis [1]

Cardiovascular

Angina [1]
Flushing [1]

Other

Application-site burning [1]
Cough [1]
Death [4]
Fibrosis [1]
Gingivitis [1]
Hypersensitivity [2]
Mucosal bleeding [1]
Pain [5]
Tooth pigmentation [1]

CARAWAY

Scientific names: *Apium carvi; Carum carvi*
Family: Apiaceae Umbelliferae
Trade and other common names: Caraway seed; Carvene; Kummel
Category: Analgesic; Anti-inflammatory; Antimicrobial; Antineoplastic; Antipyretic; Carminative; Stimulant
Purported indications and other uses: Hypotensive, dyspepsia, hysteria, tonic, stomachic. flatulent indigestion, flatulent colic of infants, fragrance, flavoring in foods, toothpaste, and cosmetics
Half-life: N/A

Reactions

Skin
  Adverse effects (sic) [2]
  Allergic reactions (sic) [1]
  Dermatitis [1]
  Urticaria [1]

Eyes
  Rhinoconjunctivitis [1]

Other
  Anaphylactoid reactions [1]
  Cough [1]
  Hypersensitivity [1]
  Sensitivity [1]

CARBAMAZEPINE

Trade names: Carbatrol; Epitol (Teva); Tegretol (Novartis)
Other common trade names: *Apo-Carbamazepine; Atreol; Foxsalepsin; Kodapan; Lexin; Mazepine; Sirtal; Tegretol XR; Teril; Timonil*
Indications: Epilepsy, pain or trigeminal neuralgia
Category: Anticonvulsant; Antimanic; Antineuralgic; Antipsychotic
Half-life: 18–55 hours
Clinically important, potentially hazardous interactions with: acetylcysteine, adenosine, aprepitant, aripiprazole, caffeine, charcoal, clarithromycin, clorazepate, clozapine, delavirdine, diltiazem, doxacurium, erythromycin, felodipine, fosamprenavir, imatinib, influenza vaccines, midazolam, solifenacin, st john's wort, telithromycin, troleandomycin, verapamil, voriconazole

Reactions

Skin
  Acne keloid [1]
  Acute generalized exanthematous
    pustulosis (AGEP) [5]
  Adverse effects (sic) [1]
  Allergic reactions (sic) [5]
  Angioedema (<1%) [4]

Anticonvulsant hypersensitivity syndrome
  [8]
Bullous eruption (<1%) [4]
Collagen disease [1]
Dermatitis [7]
Diaphoresis (1–10%)
Eczema [2]

Edema
Eosinophilic pustular folliculitis (Ofuji's disease) [1]
Epidermolysis bullosa [1]
Erythema (sheet-like)
Erythema [1]
Erythema multiforme [17]
Erythema nodosum (<1%)
Erythroderma [12]
Exanthems (>5%) [25]
Exfoliative dermatitis [22]
Facial edema [1]
Fixed eruption (<1%) [9]
Lichenoid eruption [6]
Linear IgA dermatosis [1]
Lupus erythematosus [29]
Lymphoma [2]
Mucocutaneous lymph node syndrome (Kawasaki syndrome) [2]
Mycosis fungoides [3]
Pemphigus [1]
Peripheral edema [2]
Petechiae [1]
Photosensitivity [9]
Pigmentation
Pruritus (<1%) [6]
Pseudo-mycosis fungoides [1]
Psoriasis [1]
Purpura [8]
Pustules [5]
Rash (sic) (>10%) [14]
Schamberg's disease
Side effects (sic) [2]
Stevens–Johnson syndrome (1–10%) [32]
Toxic epidermal necrolysis (1–10%) [37]
Toxic pustuloderma (probably AGEP [ed]) [3]
Toxic-allergic shock [1]
Toxicoderma [1]
Urticaria [12]
Vasculitis [5]

Hair
Hair – alopecia [6]

Nails
Nails – discoloration (bluish-black) [1]
Nails – hypoplasia [1]
Nails – lichen planus [1]
Nails – loss [1]
Nails – onychomadesis [1]

Eyes
Dyschromatopsia [1]
Periorbital edema [1]

Cardiovascular
Bradycardia [3]
Coronary artery disorders [1]
Tachycardia [1]

Other
Acute intermittent porphyria [5]
Death [1]
DRESS syndrome [5]
Dysgeusia [1]
Fetal anticonvulsant syndrome [1]
Glossitis
Headache
Hypersensitivity [47]
Lymphoproliferative disease [5]
Mania [1]
Mucocutaneous eruption [4]
Oral lichenoid eruption [1]
Oral mucosal eruption [1]
Oral ulceration [2]
Porphyria cutanea tarda [1]
Porphyria variegata [1]
Pseudolymphoma [15]
Rhabdomyolysis [1]
Seizures [2]
Serum sickness [1]
Stomatitis
test
Thrombophlebitis
Tinnitus
Tongue ulceration [2]
Xerostomia

CARBIDOPA (See LEVODOPA)

CARISOPRODOL

Synonyms: carisoprodate; isobamate
Trade name: Soma (MedPointe)
Other common trade names: *Artifar; Carisoma; Myolax; Sanoma; Sodol; Somadril; Soridol*
Indications: Painful musculoskeletal disorders
Category: Skeletal muscle relaxant
Half-life: 4–6 hours
Clinically important, potentially hazardous interactions with: eucalyptus

Reactions

Skin
  Angioedema (1–10%)
  Diaphoresis [1]
  Edema [1]
  Erythema multiforme (<1%)
  Exanthems [1]
  Fixed eruption (<1%) [2]
  Photosensitivity [1]
  Pruritus (<1%)
  Rash (sic) (<1%)
  Urticaria (<1%) [2]

Cardiovascular
  Flushing (1–10%)

Other
  Anaphylactoid reactions
  Headache
  Paresthesias [1]
  Pseudoporphyria [1]
  Tinnitus
  Trembling (1–10%)
  Xerostomia [1]

CELECOXIB

Trade name: Celebrex (Pfizer)
Indications: Osteoarthritis, rheumatoid arthritis
Category: NSAID Cox-2 inhibitor
Half-life: 11 hours

Reactions

Skin
  Acute febrile neutrophilic dermatosis
    (Sweet's syndrome) [1]
  Allergic reactions (sic) (<2%)
  Angioedema [2]
  Bacterial infections (<2%)
  Bullous eruption [1]
  Candidiasis (<2%) [1]
  Dermatitis (<2%)

  Diaphoresis (<2%)
  Edema (<2%)
  Erythema [1]
  Erythema multiforme [1]
  Exanthems (<2%) [10]
  Exfoliative dermatitis [1]
  Facial edema (<2%)
  Fixed eruption [1]
  Herpes simplex (<2%)

Herpes zoster (<2%)
Infections (<2%)
Lupus [1]
Nodular eruption (<2%)
Peripheral edema (2.1%) [4]
Photoallergic reaction [1]
Photosensitivity (<2%) [1]
Pruritus (<2%) [1]
Psoriasis (palmoplantar) [1]
Purpura [1]
Pustules [1]
Rash (sic) (2.2%)
Stevens–Johnson syndrome [1]
Toxic epidermal necrolysis [5]
Urticaria (<2%) [2]
Vasculitis [3]
Viral infections (<2%)
Xerosis (<2%)

Hair
Hair – alopecia (<2%)

Nails
Nails – changes (sic) (<2%)

Eyes
Visual disturbances [2]

Hematopoietic
Ecchymoses (<2%)

Cardiovascular
Cardiac failure [1]
Hot flashes (<2%)
Myocardial infarction [2]
Stroke [1]
Torsades de pointes [1]

Other
Anaphylactoid reactions [4]
Application-site cellulitis (<2%)
Application-site reactions (<2%)
Death [3]
Dysgeusia (<2%)
Hyperesthesia (<2%)
Hypersensitivity [2]
Mastodynia (<2%)
Myalgia (<2%)
Paresthesias (<2%)
Pseudoporphyria [1]
Stomatitis (<2%)
Tendinitis (<2%)
Thrombophlebitis (<0.1%)
Tooth disorder (sic) (<2%)
Vaginitis (<2%)
Vulvovaginal candidiasis (<2%)
Xerostomia (<2%)

*Note: Celecoxib is a sulfonamide and can be absorbed systemically. Sulfonamides can produce severe, possibly fatal, reactions such as toxic epidermal necrolysis and Stevens–Johnson syndrome

CEVIMELINE

Trade name: Exovac
Indications: Sicca syndrome in patients with Sjøgren's syndrome
Category: Cholinergic; Muscarinic agonist
Half-life: 3–4 hours

Reactions

Skin
Allergic reactions (sic) (1–10%)
Bullous eruption (<1%)
Dermatitis (<1%)
Diaphoresis (20%)

Eczema (<1%)
Edema (1–10%)
Exanthems (1–10%)
Flu-like syndrome (1–10%)
Fungal dermatitis (1–10%)

Genital pruritus (<1%)
Peripheral edema (1–10%)
Photosensitivity (<1%)
Pruritus (1–10%)
Rash (sic) (4%)
Ulcerations (<1%)
Vasculitis (<1%)
Xerosis (<1%)

Hair
Hair – alopecia (<1%)

Cardiovascular
Hot flashes (2%)

Other
Dysgeusia (<1%)
Gingival hypertrophy (<1%)

Headache
Hyperesthesia (1–10%)
Myalgia (1–10%)
Paresthesias (<1%)
Parosmia (<1%)
Sialorrhea (2%)
Stomatitis (<1%)
Tendinitis (<1%)
Thrombophlebitis (<1%)
Tongue pigmentation (<1%)
Tongue ulceration (<1%)
Tooth disorder (sic) (1–10%)
Tremor (1–10%)
Ulcerative stomatitis (1–10%)
Vaginitis (1–10%)
Xerostomia (1–10%)

CHAMOMILE

Scientific names: *Chamomilla recutita; Matricaria chamomilla; Matricaria recutita*
Family: Asteraceae; Compositae
Trade and other common names: Camomile; German Chamomile; Manzanilla; Pin Heads
Category: Sedative; Stomachic
Purported indications and other uses: Flatulence, travel sickness, nervous diarrhea, restlessness, menstrual cramps, hemorrhoids, mastitis, leg ulcers, inflammation of the respiratory tract. Used in flavoring, cosmetics, soaps and mouthwashes
Half-life: N/A
Clinically important, potentially hazardous interactions with: warfarin

Reactions

Skin
Allergic reactions (sic) (to those allergic to ragweed, marigolds, daisies)
Dermatitis [3]
Irritation

Sensitization [1]

Other
Anaphylactoid reactions [2]
Hypersensitivity

CHLOROQUINE

Trade name: Aralen (Sanofi-Aventis)
Other common trade names: *Avloclor; Chlorquin; Emquin; Heliopar; Lagaquin; Malarivon*
Indications: Malaria, rheumatoid arthritis, lupus erythematosus
Category: Antimalarial; Antiprotozoal; Antirheumatic; Lupus erythematosus suppressant
Half-life: 3–5 days
Clinically important, potentially hazardous interactions with: acitretin, antacids, cholestyramine, dapsone, furazolidone, hydroxychloroquine, methotrexate, methoxsalen, penicillamine, sulfonamides

---

Reactions

Skin
   Acute generalized exanthematous
      pustulosis (AGEP) [1]
   Angioedema (<1%) [1]
   Bullous pemphigoid [1]
   Dermatitis [2]
   Desquamation [1]
   Ephelides [1]
   Erythema annulare centrifugum [2]
   Erythema multiforme (<1%)
   Erythroderma [3]
   Exanthems (1–5%) [3]
   Exfoliative dermatitis [4]
   Fixed eruption (<1%)
   Lichenoid eruption [6]
   Photosensitivity [8]
   Pigmentation [10]
   Pruritus [31]
   Psoriasis [15]
   Pustular psoriasis [4]
   Pustules [1]
   Stevens–Johnson syndrome [4]
   Toxic epidermal necrolysis (<1%) [5]
   Urticaria [4]
   Vasculitis
   Vitiligo [8]

Hair
   Hair – alopecia

Hair – pigmentation (<1%) [8]
Hair – poliosis [3]

Nails
   Nails – discoloration [1]
   Nails – pigmentation [2]
   Nails – shoreline [1]

Eyes
   Ocular toxicity [1]

Cardiovascular
   QT prolongation [1]
   Tachycardia [1]

Other
   Acute intermittent porphyria [1]
   Death
   Gingival pigmentation [1]
   Headache
   Myalgia [2]
   Necrotizing vasculitis [1]
   Oral pigmentation [7]
   Oral ulceration [1]
   Porphyria [7]
   Porphyria cutanea tarda [1]
   Seizures [1]
   Stomatitis (<1%)
   Stomatopyrosis
   Tinnitus

CHLORZOXAZONE

Trade names: Paraflex (Ortho-McNeil); Parafon Forte DSC (Ortho-McNeil)
Other common trade names: *Escoflex; Flexaphen; Klorzoxazon; Muscol; Prolax; Remular-S; Solaxin*
Indications: Painful musculoskeletal conditions
Category: Skeletal muscle relaxant
Half-life: 1–2 hours

Reactions

Skin
  Acute generalized exanthematous
    pustulosis (AGEP) [1]
  Angioedema (1–10%)
  Erythema multiforme (<1%) [1]
  Exanthems
  Petechiae
  Pruritus
  Rash (sic) (<1%)
  Urticaria (<1%)
  Vasculitis [1]

Hematopoietic
  Ecchymoses

Cardiovascular
  Flushing (1–10%)

Other
  Anaphylactoid reactions
  Hypersensitivity
  Trembling (1–10%)

CHONDROITIN

Scientific names: *chondroitin 4- and 6-sulfate; Chondroitin 4-sulfate*
Family: None
Trade and other common names: CDS; Chondroitin Sulfate C; CSA; CSC; GAG
Category: Food supplement
Purported indications and other uses: Osteoarthritis (often with glucosamine), ischemic heart disease, osteoporosis, hyperlipidemia, keratoconjunctivitis, agent in cataract surgery
Half-life: N/A

Reactions

Skin
  Allergic reactions (sic)
  Peripheral edema

Hair
  Hair – alopecia

Eyes
  Eyelid edema [1]

CIMETIDINE

Trade name: Tagamet (GSK)
Other common trade names: *Apo-Cimetidine; Azucimet; Blocan; Cimedine; Cimehexal; Ciuk; Dyspamet; Novocimetine; Nu-Cimet; Peptol; Stomedine; Ulcedine; Zymerol*
Indications: Duodenal ulcer
Category: Antihistamine H$_2$-blocker
Half-life: 2 hours
Clinically important, potentially hazardous interactions with: alfuzosin, aminophylline, anisindione, anticoagulants, buprenorphine, butorphanol, caffeine, carmustine, dicumarol, dofetilide, duloxetine, epirubicin, fentanyl, floxuridine, fluorouracil, galantamine, hydromorphone, itraconazole, ketoconazole, lidocaine, midazolam, morphine, narcotic analgesics, oxycodone, pentazocine, phenytoin, propranolol, sufentanil, theophylline, warfarin, xanthines

Reactions

Skin
  Acne
  Angioedema (<1%) [3]
  Baboon syndrome [1]
  Erythema annulare centrifugum [2]
  Erythema multiforme (<1%) [5]
  Erythroderma
  Erythrosis-like lesions [1]
  Exanthems [3]
  Exfoliative dermatitis [2]
  Fixed eruption [2]
  Ichthyosis [1]
  Id reaction [1]
  Lupus erythematosus [2]
  Pruritus (<1%) [6]
  Psoriasis [6]
  Purpura
  Pustular psoriasis [1]
  Rash (sic) (<2%) [1]
  Seborrheic dermatitis [1]
  Side effects (sic) (0.4%) [1]

  Stevens–Johnson syndrome [3]
  Toxic dermatitis [1]
  Toxic epidermal necrolysis (<1%) [2]
  Urticaria [6]
  Vasculitis [3]
  Xerosis [1]

Hair
  Hair – alopecia [4]

Other
  Anaphylactoid reactions [1]
  Galactorrhea [1]
  Gynecomastia (<1%) [9]
  Headache
  Hypersensitivity [3]
  Injection-site pain
  Myalgia [2]
  Porphyria [1]
  Pseudolymphoma [2]
  Xerostomia

CISATRACURIUM

Trade name: Nimbex (Abbott)
Indications: Adjunct to general anesthesia, relaxes skeletal muscle
Category: Nondepolarizing neuromuscular blocker (skeletal muscle relaxant)
Half-life: 22 minutes
Clinically important, potentially hazardous interactions with: aminoglycosides, clindamycin, cyclopropane, enflurane, halothane, isoflurane, methoxyflurane, piperacillin

---
Reactions

Skin
  Rash (sic) (0.1%)

Cardiovascular
  Flushing (0.2%)

Other
  Anaphylactoid reactions [7]
  Hypersensitivity
  Myalgia [1]

CLIDINIUM

Trade names: Librax (Valeant); Quarzan
Other common trade names: *Bralix; Diporax; Epirax; Libraxin; Librocol; Nirvaxal; Spasmoten*
Indications: Duodenal and gastric ulcers
Category: Anticholinergic
Half-life: N/A
Clinically important, potentially hazardous interactions with: anticholinergics, arbutamine

Librax is clidinium and chlordiazepoxide (see chlordiazepoxide)

Reactions

Skin
  Hypohidrosis
  Purpura [1]
  Urticaria

Cardiovascular
  Flushing

Other
  Ageusia
  Anaphylactoid reactions
  Dysgeusia
  Xerostomia

CLONAZEPAM

Trade name: Klonopin (Roche)
Other common trade names: *Clonex; Iktorivil; Landsen; Lonazep; Rivotril*
Indications: Petit mal and myoclonic seizures
Category: Benzodiazepine anticonvulsant
Half-life: 18–50 hours
Clinically important, potentially hazardous interactions with: amprenavir, chlorpheniramine, clarithromycin, efavirenz, esomeprazole, imatinib, indinavir, nelfinavir, oxycodone

---

Reactions

Skin
  Allergic reactions (sic) (1–10%)
  Angioedema [1]
  Dermatitis (1–10%)
  Diaphoresis (>10%)
  Erythema multiforme [1]
  Exanthems [1]
  Facial edema
  Hypermelanosis [1]
  Peripheral edema
  Pruritus
  Pseudo-mycosis fungoides [1]
  Purpura [1]
  Rash (sic) (>10%)
  Urticaria

Hair
  Hair – alopecia [1]
  Hair – hirsutism

Other
  Black tongue [1]
  Burning mouth syndrome [1]
  Death [1]
  Dysgeusia [1]
  Gingivitis
  Headache
  Injection-site phlebitis
  Injection-site thrombosis
  Oral mucosal eruption [1]
  Oral ulceration
  Paresthesias
  Pseudolymphoma [2]
  Sialopenia (>10%)
  Sialorrhea (1–10%)
  Xerostomia (>10%) [1]

CLONIDINE

Trade names: Catapres (Boehringer Ingelheim); Combivent (Boehringer Ingelheim)
Other common trade names: *Barclyd; Catapresan; Daipres; Dixarit; Duraclon; Haemiton; Nu-Clonidine; Sulmidine*
Indications: Hypertension
Category: Alpha-2-adrenoceptor blocker; Antihypertensive
Half-life: 6–24 hours
Clinically important, potentially hazardous interactions with: acebutolol, amitriptyline, amoxapine, atenolol, betaxolol, carteolol, clomipramine, desipramine, doxepin, esmolol, imipramine, metoprolol, nadolol, nortriptyline, penbutolol, pindolol, propranolol, protriptyline, timolol, tricyclic antidepressants, trimipramine, verapamil

Combipres is clonidine and chlorthalidone

Reactions

Skin

Angioedema (<1%) [1]
Depigmentation [2]
Dermatitis (from patch) (20%) [23]
Diaphoresis [1]
Eczema [2]
Edema
Erythema [2]
Exanthems
Excoriations [1]
Herpes simplex [1]
Irritation (from patch) [1]
Lupus erythematosus [4]
Pemphigus (anogenital and cicatricial) [1]
Peripheral edema
Pigmentation [2]
Pityriasis rosea [2]
Pruritus (>5%) [5]
Psoriasis [1]
Rash (sic) (1–10%) [1]
Raynaud's phenomenon (<1%)
Scaling [1]
Ulcerations (1–10%)
Urticaria (<1%)
Vesiculation [1]

Hair

Hair – alopecia (<1%)

Cardiovascular

Bradycardia [7]
Hypotension [5]

Other

Acute intermittent porphyria
Application-site vesicles [1]
Dysgeusia (from patch)
Gynecomastia (<1%)
Headache
Hyperesthesia (1–10%)
Immune complex disease [1]
Induration [1]
Pseudolymphoma [1]
Seizures [1]
Xerostomia (40%) [7]

CLOPIDOGREL

Trade name: Plavix (Bristol-Myers Squibb) (Sanofi-Aventis)
Indications: Atherosclerotic events
Category: Antiplatelet (thienopyridine derivative)
Half-life: ~8 hours
Clinically important, potentially hazardous interactions with: anisindione, anticoagulants, dicumarol, fondaparinux, warfarin

Reactions

Skin
  Allergic reactions (sic) (1–2.5%)
  Angioedema [1]
  Bullous eruption (1–2.5%)
  Cellulitis [1]
  Eczema (1–2.5%)
  Edema (3–5%)
  Exanthems (1–2.5%) [2]
  Flu-like syndrome (7.5%)
  Lichenoid eruption (photosensitive) [1]
  Photosensitivity (lichenoid) [1]
  Pruritus (3.3%) [1]
  Purpura (5.3%) [8]
  Rash (sic) (4.2%)
  Toxic dermatitis [1]
  Ulcerations (1–2.5%)
  Urticaria (1–2.5%) [1]

Eyes
  Ocular hemorrhage [1]

Hematopoietic
  Ecchymoses [1]
  Neutropenia [1]
  Thrombocytopenic purpura [10]

Cardiovascular
  Atrial fibrillation [1]

Other
  Ageusia [1]
  Fever [1]
  Headache
  Hyperesthesia (1–2.5%)
  Hypersensitivity [1]
  Paresthesias (1–2.5%)
  Rhabdomyolysis [1]

CLORAZEPATE

Trade name: Tranxene (Ovation) (Abbott)
Other common trade names: *Gen-XENE; Novoclopate; Transene; Tranxal; Tranxen; Tranxilen; Tranxilium*
Indications: Anxiety and panic disorders
Category: Anxiolytic ; Benzodiazepine sedative-hypnotic
Half-life: 48–96 hours
Clinically important, potentially hazardous interactions with: amprenavir, antacids, carbamazepine, carmustine, chlorpheniramine, clarithromycin, efavirenz, esomeprazole, imatinib, indinavir, itraconazole, ketoconazole, MAO inhibitors, midazolam, moclobemide, nelfinavir, phenytoin, sucralfate, theophylline, warfarin

---
Reactions

Skin
  Dermatitis (1–10%)
  Diaphoresis (>10%)
  Exanthems [1]
  Photosensitivity [1]
  Pruritus
  Purpura
  Rash (sic) (>10%)
  Urticaria [1]
  Vasculitis [1]
  Vesiculation [1]

Nails
  Nails – photo-onycholysis [1]

Other
  Headache
  Oral ulceration
  Paresthesias
  Porphyria [1]
  Sialopenia (>10%)
  Sialorrhea (1–10%)
  Tremor
  Xerostomia (>10%)

CODEINE

Synonym: methylmorphine
Trade names: Calcidrine; Cheracol; Guaituss AC; Halotussin (Watson); Novahistine DH; Nucofed (Monarch); Robitussin AC (Wyeth); Tussar-2; Tussi-Organidin (MedPointe)
Other common trade names: *Actacode; Codicept; Codiforton; Paveral; Solcodein; Tricodein*
Indications: Pain, cough suppressant
Category: Antitussive; Opioid (narcotic) analgesic
Half-life: 2.5–4 hours
Clinically important, potentially hazardous interactions with: alcohol, CNS depressants, MAO inhibitors, **raspberry leaf**

Reactions

Skin
  Acute generalized exanthematous
    pustulosis (AGEP) [1]

Angioedema [2]
Bullous eruption [1]
Dermatitis [2]

Diaphoresis
Edema [1]
Erythema multiforme (<1%) [4]
Erythema nodosum (<1%) [1]
Exanthems [6]
Exfoliative dermatitis [1]
Facial edema
Fixed eruption (<1%) [6]
Photo-recall (sunlight and electronic beam)
 [1]
Pityriasis rosea [1]
Pruritus (<1%) [3]
Rash (sic) (1–10%) [1]
Toxic epidermal necrolysis (<1%) [2]
Urticaria (1–10%) [7]

Nails
 Nails – shoreline [1]

Cardiovascular
 Flushing [1]

Other
 Anaphylactoid reactions
 Dysgeusia
 Headache
 Injection-site pain (1–10%)
 Oral ulceration
 Paresthesias
 Priapism [1]
 Seizures [1]
 Trembling (<1%)
 Xerostomia (1–10%)

COENZYME Q-10

Scientific names: *Mitoquinone; Ubidecarenone; Ubiquinone*
Family: None
Trade and other common names: Co Q10; Co-Q10; CoQ; CoQ-10; Q10
Category: Food supplement
Purported indications and other uses: Congestive heart failure, angina, diabetes, hypertension, breast cancer, increasing exercise tolerance, muscular dystrophy, chronic fatigue
Half-life: N/A
Clinically important, potentially hazardous interactions with: warfarin

Note: CoQ-10 was first identified in 1957. It is widely used in Japan where millions of Japanese patients receive CoQ-10 as part of their treatment for congestive heart failure

Reactions

None

COLCHICINE

Trade name: ColBenemid
Other common trade names: *Cochiquim; Colchineos; Colgout; Goutnil; Kolkicin; Konicine*
Indications: Gouty arthritis
Category: Antigout anti-inflammatory; Uricosuric
Half-life: 20 minutes
Clinically important, potentially hazardous interactions with: clarithromycin, erythromycin, telithromycin, troleandomycin

ColBenemid is colchicine and probenecid

*Note: ColBenemid is colchicine and probenecid

Reactions

Skin
  Allergic reactions (sic) [1]
  Angioedema
  Behçet's disease [1]
  Bullous eruption (<1%) [1]
  Erythema nodosum [1]
  Erythroderma [1]
  Exanthems
  Fixed eruption [1]
  Lichenoid eruption [1]
  Necrosis
  Photosensitivity [1]
  Pruritus (<1%) [2]
  Purpura
  Pyoderma [1]
  Rash (sic) (<1%)
  Side effects (sic) (14%) [1]
  Staphylococcal scalded skin syndrome [2]
  Toxic epidermal necrolysis [3]

  Urticaria [1]
  Vasculitis [2]
  Vesiculation (palms) [1]

Hair
  Hair – alopecia (1–10%) [6]

Cardiovascular
  Flushing

Other
  Abdominal pain [1]
  Anaphylactoid reactions
  Death [2]
  Fever [1]
  Hypersensitivity
  Injection-site thrombophlebitis
  Musculoskeletal pain [1]
  Myalgia (<1%) [10]
  Porphyria cutanea tarda [1]
  Rhabdomyolysis [6]

*Note: Colchicine, by itself, is generic

COMFREY

Scientific names: *Symphytum asperum; Symphytum officinale; Symphytum x uplandicum; Symphytum. peregrinum*

Family: Boraginaceae

Trade and other common names: Ass ear; Blackwort; Boneset ; Bruisewort; consolida; consormol; consound; gum plant; knitback; Knitback; Knitbone; nipbone; Russian comfrey; Slippery Root; Wallwort

Category: Carminative

Purported indications and other uses: Leaf: Gastric and duodenal ulcer, rheumatic pain, gout, arthritis. Topical: poultice for bruises, sprains, athlete's foot, crural ulcers, mastitis, varicose ulcers. **Root:** Gastric and duodenal ulcers, hematemesis, colitis, diarrhea. Topical: ulcers, wounds, fractures, hernia

Half-life: N/A

Clinically important, potentially hazardous interactions with: eucalyptus

---

Reactions

Other
  Budd–Chiari syndrome [3]
  Death [2]

Toxicity [1]
Tumors [1]

Note: The FDA warns that comfrey contains pyrrolizidine alkaloids that can cause cirrhosis and liver failure when taken orally in high doses. It is banned in Germany and Canada. Topical application is safer and more effective; allantoin in comfrey stimulates cell proliferation, accelerating wound healing

CORTICOSTEROIDS

Generic names:

Aiclometasone [Al]
  Trade name: Aclovate (GSK)
    Topical
Amcinonide [A]
  Trade name: Cyclocort (Fujisawa)
    Topical
Beclomethasone [Be]
  Trade names: Beclovent (GSK),
    Vanceril (Schering), Beconase
    (GSK), Vancenase (Schering)
    Systemic
Betamethasone [B]
  Trade names: Celestone (Schering),
    Betaderm (Roaco), Diprosone
    (Schering), Luxiq (Connetics)
    Systemic/Topical

Budesonide [Bu]
  Trade name: Rhinocort
    (AstraZeneca)
    Systemic
Clobetasol
  Trade names: Temovate (GSK),
    Embeline (HealthPoint), Olux
    (Connetics)
    Topical/Systemic
Cortisone [C]
    Systemic
Desonide
  Trade name: DesOwen (Galderma)
    Topical
Desoximetasone
  Trade name: Topicort (Medicis)
    Topical

Dexamethasone [D]
    Trade name: Decadron [Merck]
        Systemic/Topical
Fludrocortisone
    Trade name: Florinef (Apothecon)
        Systemic
Flumetasone
    Trade names: Locacorten (Paladin),
        Locasalen (Bioglan)
        Topical
Flunisolide
    Trade names: Aerobid (Forest),
        Nasalide (Ivax)
        Systemic
Fluocinolone
    Trade names: Capex (Galderma),
        Synalar (Medicis), Synemol
        (Medicis)
        Topical
Fluocinonide
    Topical
Flurandrenolide
    Trade name: Cordan
        Topical
Fluticasone [Ft]
    Trade names: Cutivate (GSK);
        Flonase (GSK)
        Topical/Systemic
Halcinonide
    Trade name: Halog (BMS)
        Topical
Halobetasol
    Trade name: Ultravate (BMS)
        Topical

Halomethasone
    Trade name: Sicorten
        Topical
Hydrocortisone [H]
    Trade names: Hytone (Dermik);
        Cortef (Pfizer); Solu-Cortef
        (Pfizer)
        Systemic/Topical
Methylprednisolone [M]
    Trade names: Medrol (Pfizer); Depo-
        Medrol (Pfizer); Solu-Medrol
        (Pfizer)
        Systemic
Mometasone
    Trade names: Elocon (Schering);
        Elocom (Schering)
        Topical
Prednicarbate
    Trade name: Dermatop (Dermik)
        Topical
Prednisolone [Prl]
    Trade name: Delta-Cortef (Pfizer)
Prednisone [Pr]
    Trade names: Deltasone (Pfizer);
        Orasone
        Systemic
Triamcinolone [T]
    Trade names: Aristocort (Fujisawa);
        Azmacort (Kos); Kenalog
        Topical/Systemic
Tixocortol [Tx]
    Trade name: (not available in USA)
        Topical

Category: Anti-inflammatory

Clinically important, potentially hazardous interactions with: acitretin, aldesleukin, anticholinesterases, cascara, cyclosporine, didanosine, diltiazem, doxycycline, **echinacea**, edrophonium, **grapefruit juice**, imatinib, isotretinoin, **mistletoe**, mycophenolate, physostigmine, rifabutin, rifampin, rifapentine, **smallpox vaccine**, tetracycline, **varicella vaccine**

	Reactions

Skin
  Acanthosis nigricans [3]
  Acne [7]

Acute generalized exanthematous
  pustulosis (AGEP) [1]
Allergic reactions (sic) [4]

Angioedema [2]
Atrophy [8]
Bacterial infections
Bruising [1]
Bullous eruption [1]
Calcification [1]
Candidiasis [1]
Cellulitis [1]
Depigmentation [3]
Dermatitis [13]
Dermatofibromas [2]
Diaphoresis [1]
Eczema [4]
Erythema (diffuse and widespread) [4]
Erythema multiforme [1]
Exanthems [3]
Facial edema [2]
Facial erythema
Fixed eruption [1]
Fungal dermatitis
Herpes simplex
Herpes zoster
Infections [1]
Kaposi's sarcoma [4]
Leucoderma acquisitum [1]
Linear atrophy [4]
Linear hypopigmentation [6]
Lupus erythematosus [1]
Necrosis [1]
Perianal ulcerations [1]
Perioral dermatitis [2]
Photosensitivity [1]
Pigmentation [3]
Pityriasis rosea [1]
Porokeratosis [1]
Pruritus [5]
Pseudoxanthoma elasticum [1]
Purpura [5]
Pustular psoriasis [1]
Rash (sic) [1]
Staphylococcal scalded skin syndrome [1]
Striae [3]
Telangiectasia [3]
Thinning [3]

Urticaria [9]
Vasculitis [4]
Viral infections

Hair
Hair – alopecia [1]
Hair – hirsutism
Hair – hypertrichosis [2]

Eyes
Chorioretinopathy [1]
Uveitis [1]

Hematopoietic
Ecchymoses [4]

Cardiovascular
Coronary artery disorders [1]
Flushing [2]

Other
Anaphylactoid reactions [12]
Anxiety [1]
Black tongue
Buffalo hump [1]
Dementia [1]
Depression [1]
Embolia cutis medicamentosa (Nicolau syndrome) [1]
Fever [1]
Hypersensitivity [3]
Impaired wound healing [1]
Injection-site aseptic necrosis
Injection-site lipoatrophy [5]
Mania [1]
Mood changes (n = 8) [1]
Moon face [1]
Mucocutaneous eruption [1]
Myalgia [8]
Oral candidiasis [3]
Osteopenia [1]
Panniculitis [1]
Pneumonia [1]
Psychosis [1]
Seizures [1]
Stomatitis [1]

CREATINE

Scientific names: *N-(aminoiminomethyl)-N methyl glycine; N-amidinosarcosine*
Family: None
Trade and other common names: Cr; Creatine monohydrate
Category: Food supplement
Purported indications and other uses: Improve exercise performance, increase muscle mass, heart failure, neuromuscular disease, cholesterol-lowering, amyotrophic lateral sclerosis (ALS), rheumatoid arthritis, cardiac surgery (IV)
Half-life: N/A

Reactions

Skin
  Acne [1]
  Facial rash (sic) [1]

Eyes
  Periorbital edema [1]

Other
  Anaphylactoid reactions [1]
  Myalgia [1]
  Polymyositis [1]
  Rhabdomyolysis [3]
  Side effects (sic) [1]

*Note: Creatine is found primarily in skeletal muscle (95%), also in heart, brain, testes & other tissues. The body synthesizes 1 to 2 grams of creatine a day

**Note: Creatine use is widespread among amateur and professional athletes including, Mark McGuire, Sammy Sosa, John Elway and others. The annual consumption of creatine in the US exceeds 10 million pounds

CYCLOBENZAPRINE

Trade name: Flexeril (McNeil) (Merck)
Other common trade names: *Benzamin; Cloben; Cyben; Flexiban; Novo-Cycloprine; Yurelax*
Indications: Muscle spasms
Category: Skeletal muscle relaxant
Half-life: 1–3 days

Reactions

Skin
  Allergic reactions (sic)
  Angioedema (<1%)
  Dermatitis (<1%)
  Diaphoresis [1]
  Facial edema (<1%)
  Photosensitivity
  Pruritus (<1%)
  Purpura
  Rash (sic) (<1%)
  Urticaria (<1%)

Hair
  Hair – alopecia

Cardiovascular
  Flushing

Other
  Ageusia (<1%)

Anaphylactoid reactions (<1%)
Dysgeusia (3%)
Galactorrhea
Gynecomastia
Headache
Paresthesias (<1%)

Stomatitis
Tinnitus
Tongue edema (<1%)
Tongue pigmentation
Xerostomia (27%) [2]

CYPROHEPTADINE

Trade names: Ciplactin; Ciproral; Nuran; Periactine; Periactinol; Peritol; Sigloton
Indications: Allergic rhinitis, urticaria
Category: Antihistamine H$_1$-blocker
Half-life: 1–4 hours
Clinically important, potentially hazardous interactions with: anticholinergics, MAO inhibitors, phenelzine, tranylcypromine

Reactions

Skin
  Allergic reactions (sic) (<1%)
  Angioedema (<1%)
  Dermatitis [1]
  Diaphoresis
  Edema (<1%)
  Erythema
  Exanthems [1]
  Lichenoid eruption [1]
  Lupus erythematosus
  Peripheral edema
  Photosensitivity [1]
  Purpura
  Rash (sic) (<1%)

Urticaria
Vasculitis [1]

Cardiovascular
  Flushing

Other
  Anaphylactoid reactions
  Dysgeusia [1]
  Myalgia (<1%)
  Paresthesias (<1%)
  Tinnitus
  Xerostomia (1–10%) [2]

DANTROLENE

Trade name: Dantrium (Procter & Gamble)
Other common trade names: *Dantamacrin; Dantrolen*
Indications: Spasticity, malignant hyperthermia
Category: Skeletal muscle relaxant
Half-life: 8.7 hours
Clinically important, potentially hazardous interactions with: verapamil

Reactions

Skin
  Acne [2]
  Chills (1–10%)
  Dermatitis
  Diaphoresis
  Erythema
  Exanthems [1]
  Photosensitivity
  Pruritus
  Rash (sic) (>10%)
  Urticaria

Hair
  Hair – hypertrichosis

Other
  Anaphylactoid reactions
  Dysgeusia
  Headache
  Malignant lymphoma [1]
  Myalgia
  Thrombophlebitis
  Tremor

DESFLURANE

Trade name: Suprane (Baxter)
Other common trade name: *Sulorane*
Indications: Induction or maintenance of anesthesia
Category: General anesthetic
Half-life: Onset of action: 1–2 minutes
Clinically important, potentially hazardous interactions with: tramadol

Reactions

Skin
  Pruritus
  Shivering [1]

Other
  Cough (34%)

Death [1]
Malignant hyperthermia [7]
Myalgia
Pharyngitis (3–10%)

DEVIL'S CLAW

Scientific names: *Harpagophytum procumbens; Harpagophytum zeyheri*
Family: Pedaliaceae
Trade and other common names: Doloteffin; Grapple plant; Griffe du diable; Harpadol; wood spider
Category: Analgesic; Anti-inflammatory; Antioxidant; Antiviral; Diuretic
Purported indications and other uses: Oral: anorexia, arteriosclerosis, rheumatoid arthritis, GI disorders, fibromyalgia, loss of appetite, headache, fever, high cholesterol, menstrual complaints, liver and gallbladder problems. Topical: rash, ulcers
Half-life: 3–6 hours
Clinically important, potentially hazardous interactions with: anesthetics, antacids, antiarrhythmic drugs, anticoagulants, aspirin, beta blockers, digoxin, famotidine, histamine 2 blockers (e.g ranitidine), hypoglycemics, NSAIDs, ranitidine, sympathomimetics, terfenadine, warfarin

Reactions

Skin
  Adverse effects (sic) [4]

Other
  Dysgeusia [1]
  Tinnitus [1]

Note: Devil's claw stimulates stomach acid production, and should be avoided by those with stomach or duodenal ulcers. It should not be taken by people with cardiac arrhythmias or other heart problems

DICLOFENAC

Trade names: Arthrotec (Pfizer); Solaraze Gel (Doak); Voltaren (Novartis)
Other common trade names: *Allvoran; Apo-Diclo; Fenac; Galedol; Liroken; Monoflam; Nu-Diclo; Remethan; Taks; Voltarene; Voltarol*
Indications: Rheumatoid and osteoarthritis
Category: Nonsteroidal anti-inflammatory (NSAID)
Half-life: 1–2 hours
Clinically important, potentially hazardous interactions with: methotrexate, telithromycin

Arthrotec is diclofenac and misoprostol

Reactions

Skin
  Adverse effects (sic) [1]
  Allergic reactions (sic) [2]
  Angioedema (1–3%) [1]
  Bullous eruption (1–3%) [2]
  Dermatitis (1–3%) [12]

Dermatitis herpetiformis [2]
Dermatomyositis [1]
Diaphoresis (<1%)
Eczema (1–3%)
Edema
Erythema [3]

Erythema multiforme (<1%) [7]
Erythema nodosum (<1%)
Exanthems (1–5%) [6]
Exfoliative dermatitis (<1%)
Fixed eruption [1]
Lichenoid eruption [1]
Linear IgA dermatosis [5]
Lupus erythematosus
Necrosis [1]
Necrotizing fasciitis [1]
Pemphigus [1]
Peripheral edema [1]
Photoallergic reaction [1]
Photosensitivity (1–3%) [5]
Pruritus (1–10%) [6]
Pseudoreactions (sic) [1]
Psoriasis [3]
Purpura (1–3%) [2]
Purpura fulminans [1]
Pustular psoriasis [3]
Rash (sic) (>10%) [1]
Stevens–Johnson syndrome (1–3%) (1 fatal case) [2]
Toxic epidermal necrolysis [3]
Urticaria (1–3%) [6]
Vasculitis [4]

Hair
Hair – alopecia (1–3%)

Cardiovascular
Angina [1]
Arrhythmias [1]
Flushing (<1%)

Other
Acute intermittent porphyria
Anaphylactoid reactions (1–3%) [8]
Aphthous stomatitis [1]
Death [2]
Dysgeusia (1–3%)
Embolia cutis medicamentosa (Nicolau syndrome) [6]
Headache
Hypersensitivity [3]
Injection-site necrosis [1]
Injection-site pain [1]
Oral ulceration [1]
Paresthesias (<1%)
Pseudolymphoma [1]
Rhabdomyolysis [2]
Serum sickness
Still's disease [1]
Stomatitis (<1%)
Systemic reactions [1]
Tinnitus
Tongue edema (1–3%)
Xerostomia (1–3%) [1]

DICYCLOMINE

Trade names: Antispaz; Bemote; Bentyl (Axcan); Byclomine; Di-Spaz; Dibent; Neoquess; OrTyl; Spasmoject
Other common trade names: *Bentylol; Formulex; Lomine; Merbentyl; Notensyl; Panakiron; Spasmoban; Swityl*
Indications: Irritable bowel syndrome
Category: Anticholinergic; Antispasmodic
Half-life: initial: 1.8 hours; terminal: 9–10 hours
Clinically important, potentially hazardous interactions with: anticholinergics, arbutamine

Reactions

Skin
Exanthems [2]

Hypohidrosis (>10%)
Pruritus [1]

Rash (sic) (<1%) [2]
Urticaria
Xerosis (>10%)

Cardiovascular
Flushing

Other
Ageusia

Anaphylactoid reactions
Dysgeusia
Headache
Injection-site reactions (sic) (>10%)
Tremor
Xerostomia (>10%) [1]

DIFLUNISAL

Trade name: Dolobid (Merck)
Other common trade names: *Ansal; Apo-Diflunisal; Diflonid; Diflusal; Dolobis; Donobid; Fluniget; Flustar; Nu-Diflunisal*
Indications: Rheumatoid and osteoarthritis
Category: Nonsteroidal anti-inflammatory (NSAID) analgesic
Half-life: 8–12 hours
Clinically important, potentially hazardous interactions with: indomethacin

Reactions

Skin
Adverse effects (sic) [2]
Angioedema (<1%)
Bullous eruption [1]
Diaphoresis (<1%) [2]
Edema (<1%)
Erythema multiforme (<1%) [5]
Erythroderma [2]
Exanthems [4]
Exfoliative dermatitis (<1%) [1]
Fixed eruption [2]
Lichenoid eruption [1]
Peripheral edema
Photosensitivity (<1%) [1]
Pruritus (1–10%) [3]
Purpura
Rash (sic) (3–9%) [3]
Stevens–Johnson syndrome (<1%) [7]
Toxic epidermal necrolysis (<1%) [1]
Urticaria (>1%) [6]
Vasculitis (<1%)

Hair
Hair – alopecia [1]

Nails
Nails – onycholysis

Cardiovascular
Flushing (<1%)

Other
Anaphylactoid reactions (<1%)
Aphthous stomatitis
Headache
Hypersensitivity (<1%)
Oral lichen planus [1]
Oral ulceration
Paresthesias (<1%)
Pseudolymphoma [1]
Pseudoporphyria [1]
Stomatitis (<1%)
Tinnitus
Trembling (<1%)
Xerostomia [1]

DIHYDROERGOTAMINE

Trade names: D.H.E. 45 (Xcel); Migranal (Xcel)
Other common trade names: *Dergiflux; Dihydergot; Ergont; Ergovasan; Ikaran; Orstanorm; Seglor; Verladyn; Verteblan*
Indications: Prevention of vascular headaches
Category: Ergot alkaloid
Half-life: 1.3–3.9 hours
Clinically important, potentially hazardous interactions with: almotriptan, amprenavir, clarithromycin, delavirdine, efavirenz, erythromycin, fosamprenavir, indinavir, naratriptan, nelfinavir, ritonavir, rizatriptan, saquinavir, sibutramine, sumatriptan, troleandomycin, zolmitriptan

Reactions

Skin
  Edema (>10%)
  Pruritus

Cardiovascular
  Hypertension [1]

Other
  Dysgeusia

Headache
Injection-site reactions (sic)
Myalgia
Paresthesias (>10%)
Xerostomia (>10%)

DILTIAZEM

Trade names: Cardizem (Biovail); Cartia-XT; Dilacor XR (Watson); Diltia-XT; Teczem (Sanofi-Aventis); Tiazac (Forest)
Other common trade names: *Alti-Diltiazem; Britiazem; Calcicard; Deltazen; Dilrene; Diltahexal; Nu-Diltiaz; Presoken; Tiamate; Tilazem; Tildiem*
Indications: Angina, essential hypertension
Category: Antianginal; Antiarrhythmic; Calcium channel blocker
Half-life: 5–8 hours (for extended-release capsules)
Clinically important, potentially hazardous interactions with: alfuzosin, amiodarone, aprepitant, carbamazepine, corticosteroids, cyclosporine, epirubicin, erythromycin, mistletoe, simvastatin

Teczem is diltiazem and enalapril

Reactions

Skin
  Acne [1]
  Acute generalized exanthematous
    pustulosis (AGEP) [12]
  Adverse effects (sic) [1]
  Angioedema [2]

Capillaritis (Schamberg's) [1]
Dermatitis
Diaphoresis [2]
Edema (1–10%) [4]
Erythema [2]
Erythema multiforme (1–31%) [9]

Exanthems [16]
Exfoliative dermatitis (<1%) [6]
Hyperkeratosis (feet) [1]
Lichenoid eruption (photosensitive) [2]
Lupus erythematosus [5]
Palmar–plantar desquamation [1]
Peripheral edema (5–8%) [2]
Petechiae (<1%)
Photosensitivity (<1%) [11]
Pigmentation [4]
Pruritus (<1%) [7]
Psoriasis [3]
Purpura (<1%) [3]
Pustular psoriasis [1]
Pustules [2]
Rash (sic) (1.3%) [3]
Side effects (sic) [2]
Stevens–Johnson syndrome [4]
Subcorneal pustular dermatosis [2]
Thickening [2]
Toxic dermatitis [1]
Toxic epidermal necrolysis [4]
Toxic erythema [2]
Ulcerations of legs [2]
Urticaria (<1%) [4]
Vasculitis (<1%) [6]

Hair

Hair – alopecia (<1%) [2]
Hair – hirsutism [1]

Nails

Nails – dystrophy [1]

Eyes

Periorbital edema [1]

Hematopoietic

Ecchymoses (<1%)

Cardiovascular

Atrial fibrillation [1]
Bradycardia [4]
Flushing (1–10%) [5]
Hypertension [1]

Other

Dysgeusia (<1%) [1]
Erythromelalgia [1]
Fever [1]
Gingival hypertrophy (21%) [6]
Gynecomastia [1]
Headache
Hypersensitivity [1]
Lymphadenopathy [1]
Myoclonus [1]
Parageusia (<1%)
Paresthesias (<1%) [1]
Parkinsonism [2]
Pseudolymphoma [1]
Rhabdomyolysis [3]
Tinnitus
Tremor (<1%)
Xerostomia (<1%) [2]

DIVALPROEX (See VALPROIC ACID)

DOMPERIDONE

Trade names: Evoxin; Motilium (Johnson & Johnson)
Indications: Investigational antiemetic, gastroesophageal reflux disease (GERD), nausea and vomiting
Category: Peripherally-acting dopamine-2-receptor antagonist
Half-life: 7–8 hours

Note: Domperamol is domperidone & acetaminophen

Reactions

Skin
Diaphoresis
Edema
Edema of lip
Facial edema
Facial erythema
Lupus erythematosus [1]
Neuroleptic malignant syndrome (<0.1%)
 [1]
Pruritus
Rash (sic) [1]
Urticaria

Cardiovascular
QT prolongation [1]

Other
Anaphylactoid reactions
Breast changes
Death [2]
Depression [1]
Dry mucous membranes
Galactorrhea [5]
Gynecomastia [2]
Hypersensitivity
Parkinsonism [1]
Rhabdomyolysis [1]
Tremor

DONEPEZIL

Synonym: E2020
Trade name: Aricept (Eisai) (Endo)
Indications: Mild dementia of the Alzheimer's type
Category: Cholinergic ; Reversible acetylcholinesterase inhibitor for Alzheimer's disease
Half-life: 50–70 hours
Clinically important, potentially hazardous interactions with: galantamine

Reactions

Skin
Dermatitis (<1%)
Diaphoresis (>1%)
Erythema (<1%)
Facial edema (<1%)
Hyperkeratosis (<1%)
Neurodermatitis (<1%)

Neuroleptic malignant syndrome [1]
Pigmentation (<1%)
Pruritus (>1%)
Purpura (1–10%) [1]
Striae (<1%)
Ulcerations (<1%)
Urticaria (>1%)

Hair
Hair – alopecia (<1%)
Hair – hirsutism (<1%)

Eyes
Periorbital edema (<1%)

Hematopoietic
Ecchymoses (4%)

Cardiovascular
Atrial fibrillation [1]
Flushing [1]

Other
Anxiety [1]

Depression [1]
Dizziness [1]
Dysgeusia (<1%)
Fatigue [1]
Gingivitis (<1%)
Headache [1]
Paresthesias (<1%)
Rhinitis [1]
Tongue edema (<1%)
Vaginitis (<1%)
Xerostomia (<1%)

DONG QUAI

Scientific name: *Angelica sinensis (Angelica polymorpha sinensis)*
Family: Umbelliferae; Apioideae
Trade and other common names: Dang Gui; Dang Kwai; Danggui; Dong qua; Tan Kue; Tang Quai; Tank Kuei
Category: Immunostimulant; Phytoestrogen
Purported indications and other uses: Menopausal symptoms, PMS, menstrual disorders, anemia, constipation, insomnia, rheumatism, neuralgia, hypertension, hypopigmentation, psoriasis
Half-life: N/A
Clinically important, potentially hazardous interactions with: acetaminophen, dipyridamole, heparin, tamoxifen, ticlopidine, warfarin

---
Reactions

Skin
Photosensitivity
Phototoxicity

Other
Gynecomastia [2]

Note: Some recent research has questioned the efficacy of Dong Quai, and also suggested that it may be a potential carcinogen

DOXACURIUM

Trade name: Nuromax (GSK)
Indications: Neuromuscular blockade
Category: Neuromuscular blocker; Skeletal muscle relaxant
Half-life: 100–200 minutes
Clinically important, potentially hazardous interactions with: amikacin, aminoglycosides, carbamazepine, cyclopropane, enflurane, gentamicin, halothane, isoflurane, kanamycin, methoxyflurane, neomycin, piperacillin, streptomycin, tobramycin

---

Reactions

Skin   Urticaria (<1%)
  Rash (sic)

ECHINACEA

Scientific names: *Echinacea angustifolia; Echinacea pallida; Echinacea purpurea*
Family: Asteraceae; Compositae
Trade and other common names: Black Sampson; Black Susans; Comb Flower; Indian Head; Purple-Cone Flower; Snakeroot
Category: Antiseptic; Antiviral; Immunomodulator
Purported indications and other uses: Colds, upper respiratory infections, peripheral vasodilator, urinary tract infections, yeast infections, ulcers, psoriasis, herpes simplex, septicemia, boils, abscesses, rheumatism, migraine, dyspepsia, eczema, bee stings and hemorrhoids
Half-life: N/A
Clinically important, potentially hazardous interactions with: corticosteroids, cyclosporine

---

Reactions

Skin   Urticaria [2]
  Adverse effects (sic) [4]   **Other**
  Allergic reactions (sic)   Anaphylactoid reactions [3]
  Angioedema [1]   Dizziness [1]
  Bullae [1]   Hypersensitivity [2]
  Erythema nodosum [1]   Oral mucosal lesions [1]
  Rash (sic) [1]   Paresthesias
  Sensitization [1]   Sialorrhea

Note: Individuals with atopy may be more likely to experience an allergic reaction when taking Echinacea

EDROPHONIUM

Trade names: Enlon (Baxter); Tensilon (Valeant)
Indications: Myasthenia gravis diagnosis
Category: Anticholinesterase; Antidote; Neuromuscular blocker
Half-life: 1.8 hours
Clinically important, potentially hazardous interactions with: corticosteroids, galantamine

Reactions

Skin
Diaphoresis (>10%)
Rash (sic)
Urticaria

Cardiovascular
Flushing

Other
Anaphylactoid reactions
Headache
Hypersensitivity (<1%)
Sialorrhea (>10%)
Thrombophlebitis (<1%)

ELETRIPTAN

Trade name: Relpax (Pfizer)
Indications: Migraine headaches
Category: Serotonin agonist
Half-life: 4–5 hours

Reactions

Skin
Abscess (<1%)
Allergic reactions (sic) (<1%)
Candidiasis (<1%)
Chills (<1%)
Diaphoresis (<1%)
Edema (<1%)
Exanthems (<1%)
Exfoliative dermatitis (<1%)
Facial edema (<1%)
Peripheral edema (<1%)
Pigmentation (<1%)
Pruritus (<1%)
Psoriasis (<1%)
Rash (sic) (<1%)
Urticaria (<1%)
Xerosis (<1%)

Hair
Hair – alopecia

Other
Arthralgia (<1%)
Depression (<1%)
Dysgeusia (<1%)
Foetor ex ore (halitosis) (<1%)
Gingivitis (<1%)
Headache
Hyperesthesia (<1%)
Mastodynia (<1%)
Myalgia (<1%)
Paresthesias (<1%)
Parosmia (<1%)
Sialorrhea (<1%)
Stomatitis (<1%)
Tinnitus (<1%)
Tongue disorder (<1%)

Tooth disorder (sic) (<1%)   Twitching (<1%)
Tremor (<1%)   Vaginitis (<1%)

ENFLURANE

Trade name: Ethrane (Baxter)
Other common trade names: *Alyrane; Efrane; Etrane*
Indications: Maintenance of general anesthesia
Category: General anesthetic
Half-life: N/A
Clinically important, potentially hazardous interactions with: cisatracurium, doxacurium, pancuronium, rapacuronium

Reactions

Skin   **Other**
  Shivering   Rhabdomyolysis [1]
                                             Seizures [1]

ENTACAPONE

Trade name: Comtan (Novartis)
Other common trade name: *Comtess*
Indications: Parkinsonism
Category: Antiparkinsonian; Reverse COMT inhibitor
Half-life: 2.4 hours
Clinically important, potentially hazardous interactions with: MAO inhibitors, phenelzine, tranylcypromine

Reactions

Skin   Dysgeusia (1%)
  Bacterial infections (1%)   Dyskinesia (31%) [1]
  Bullous eruption [1]   Headache
  Diaphoresis (2%)   Parkinsonism (17%) [1]
  Purpura (2%)   Xerostomia (3%)

Other
  Dizziness (20%) [1]

EPHEDRA

Scientific names: *Ephedra equisetina; Ephedra intermedia; Ephedra sinica; Ephedra vulgaris*
Family: Gnetaceae
Trade and other common names: Joint Fir; Ma Huang; Popotillo; Sea Grape; Teamster's Tea; Yellow Astringent; Yellow Horse
Category: Cardiovascular stimulant; CNS stimulant
Purported indications and other uses: Bronchospasm, asthma, bronchitis, allergy, appetite suppressant, colds, flu, fever, chills, edema, headache, anhidrosis, diuretic, joint and bone pain
Half-life: N/A
Clinically important, potentially hazardous interactions with: acetazolamide, amitriptyline, caffeine, corticosteriods, ephedrine, epinephrine, guanethidine, guarana, MAO inhibitors, olmesartan, phenelzine, phenylpropanolamine, selegiline, sibutramine, sodium bicarbonate

Reactions

Skin
  Adverse effects (sic) [3]

Cardiovascular
  Flushing

Other
  Death [3]

Eosinophilia–myalgia syndrome [1]
Hypersensitivity
Seizures [4]
Side effects (sic) [1]
Tremor
Xerostomia [1]

Note: The FDA has recently banned Ephedra because of serious side effects

ESTRAMUSTINE

Trade name: Emcyt (Pfizer)
Other common trade name: *Cellmusin*
Indications: Prostate carcinoma
Category: Antineoplastic; Nitrogen mustard
Half-life: 20 hours
Clinically important, potentially hazardous interactions with: aldesleukin

Reactions

Skin
  Allergic reactions (sic) [1]
  Angioedema [1]
  Edema (>10%)
  Exanthems [1]
  Night sweats (<1%)
  Pigmentation (<1%)
  Pruritus (2%) [1]
  Purpura (3%)

  Rash (sic) (1%)
  Urticaria
  Xerosis (2%)

Hair
  Hair – alopecia (<1%)

Cardiovascular
  Flushing (1%)
  Hot flashes (<1%)

Other
Death [1]
Gynecomastia (>10%)
Injection-site thrombophlebitis (1–10%) [1]

Mastodynia (66%)
Thrombophlebitis (3%)
Tinnitus

ETANERCEPT

Trade name: Enbrel (Amgen) (Wyeth)
Indications: Rheumatoid arthritis
Category: Antiarthritic; Antirheumatic; Biologic response modifier
Half-life: 98–300 hours
Clinically important, potentially hazardous interactions with: anakinra

Reactions

Skin
Adverse effects (sic) [2]
Allergic reactions (sic) (<3%)
Cellulitis [1]
Erythema
Exanthems [2]
Herpes zoster [1]
Infections (<3%) [6]
Lupus erythematosus [12]
Lymphoma [1]
Malignancies (sic) (<3%)
Peripheral edema [1]
Pruritus [1]
Psoriasis [2]
Purpura [1]
Rash (sic) (5%) [3]
Squamous cell carcinoma (penis) [3]
Ulcerations
Upper respiratory infection [1]
Urticaria [2]
Vasculitis [8]

Hair
Hair – alopecia [1]

Eyes
Uveitis [1]

Hematopoietic
Aplastic anemia [1]

Leukopenia [1]
Neutropenia [1]
Pancytopenia [1]
Thrombocytopenia [1]

Cardiovascular
Atrial fibrillation [1]

Other
Abdominal pain [1]
Asthenia [1]
Cough [1]
Death [2]
Depression [1]
Dizziness [1]
Headache [2]
Injection-site reactions (sic) (20–40%) [20]
Lymphoproliferative disease [1]
Nodular eruption [2]
Oral ulceration [1]
Pharyngitis [1]
Polymyositis [1]
Rheumatoid nodules [1]
Rhinitis [2]
Sinusitis [1]
Thrombophlebitis [1]
Tinnitus [1]
Toxoplasmosis [1]
Tuberculosis [1]

ETHOSUXIMIDE

Trade name: Zarontin (Pfizer)
Other common trade names: *Emeside; Ethymal; Petnidan; Pyknolepsinum; Simatin; Zarondan*
Indications: Absence (petit mal) seizures
Category: Succinimide anticonvulsant
Half-life: 50–60 hours

Reactions

Skin
  Anticonvulsant hypersensitivity syndrome
    [1]
  Erythema multiforme (<1%) [1]
  Exanthems (1–5%) [2]
  Exfoliative dermatitis (<1%)
  Lupus erythematosus (>10%) [19]
  Pruritus
  Purpura [1]
  Rash (sic) (<1%)
  Raynaud's phenomenon [3]
  Side effects (sic) (3.4%) [1]
  Stevens–Johnson syndrome (>10%) [1]
  Urticaria (1–5%) [1]

Hair
  Hair – alopecia
  Hair – hirsutism

Eyes
  Periorbital edema

Other
  Acute intermittent porphyria
  Gingival hypertrophy
  Headache
  Oral ulceration
  Tongue edema

ETHOTOIN

Trade name: Peganone (Ovation)
Other common trade name: *Accenon*
Indications: Tonic–clonic (grand mal) seizures
Category: Hydantoin anticonvulsant
Half-life: 3–9 hours
Clinically important, potentially hazardous interactions with: chloramphenicol,
cyclosporine, disulfiram, dopamine, imatinib, itraconazole

Reactions

Skin
  Bullous eruption
  Fixed eruption
  Lupus erythematosus
  Purpura [1]

  Rash (sic)

Other
  Gingival hypertrophy
  Pseudolymphoma [1]

ETODOLAC

Trade name: Lodine (Wyeth)
Other common trade names: *Antilak; Ecridoxan; Edolan; Elderin; Lonine; Tedolan; Utradol; Zedolac*
Indications: Pain
Category: Nonsteroidal anti-inflammatory (NSAID)
Half-life: 7 hours
Clinically important, potentially hazardous interactions with: aspirin, methotrexate

Reactions

Skin
 Angioedema (<1%) [1]
 Bullous eruption
 Dermatitis
 Diaphoresis
 Edema
 Erythema multiforme (<1%)
 Exanthems [4]
 Exfoliative dermatitis
 Facial edema [2]
 Fixed eruption [1]
 Furunculosis [1]
 Peripheral edema [1]
 Photosensitivity [1]
 Pigmentation
 Pruritus (1–10%) [8]
 Purpura
 Rash (sic) (>10%) [5]
 Stevens–Johnson syndrome (<1%)
 Toxic epidermal necrolysis (<1%)
 Urticaria (<1%) [2]

 Vasculitis [2]
 Vesiculobullous eruption

Hair
 Hair – alopecia

Hematopoietic
 Ecchymoses

Cardiovascular
 Flushing [1]

Other
 Gingival ulceration
 Glossitis
 Gynecomastia
 Parageusia
 Paresthesias
 Sialorrhea
 Stomatitis
 Tinnitus
 Ulcerative stomatitis
 Xerostomia

EUCALYPTUS

Scientific names: *Eucalyptus bicostata; Eucalyptus fruticetorum; Eucalyptus globulus; Eucalyptus odorata; Eucalyptus pauciflora; Eucalyptus polybractea; Eucalyptus smithii*

Family: Myrtacceae

Trade and other common names: Blue gum; Blue mallee oil; Dristan Nasal Decongestant Spray; Fever tree; Gully gum oil; Listerine; Red gum; Stringy bark; Vicks VapoRub. Mentho-Lyptus (Hall) in mouthwash; toothpaste, cough drops, lozenges

Category: Anti-inflammatory; Antibacterial; Antiseptic; Antispasmodic; Diuretic; Expectorant; Stimulant

Purported indications and other uses: Asthma, Bronchitis, Cough, Croup, Fever, Joint and Muscle Pains, Nasal Congestion, Sore Throats, Rheumatism.

Flavoring, Fragrance, Toothpaste, Substances used in root canal fillings

Half-life: N/A

Clinically important, potentially hazardous interactions with: amitriptyline, borage, carisoprodol, coltsfoot, comfrey, diazepam, haloperidol, insulin, lansoprazole, nelfinavir, omeprazole, ondansetron, pantoprazole, propranolol, theophylline, verapamil

*Possible interactions, no definitive data

Reactions

Skin
  Cyanosis
  Dermatitis [1]
  Rash [1]

Eyes
  Miosis

Other
  Ataxia [2]
  Death [O]
  Dizziness
  Muscle weakness [1]
  Seizures [1]
  Toxicity
  Unconsciousness [2]

Note: [O] is oral

EVENING PRIMROSE

Scientific names: *Oenothera biennis; Oenothera muricata; Oenothera purpurata; Oenothera rubricaulis; Oenothera suaveolens*

Family: Onagraceae

Trade and other common names: EPO; Fever Plant; Gamma Linolenic Acid; GLA; Night Willow-Herb; Scabish; Sun Drop

Category: Anti-inflammatory; Essential fatty acid

Purported indications and other uses: Mastalgia, Osteoporosis, Atopic Dermatitis, Rheumatoid Arthritis, Hypercholesterolemia, Chronic Fatigue Syndrome, Neurodermatitis, Ulcerative Colitis, Irritable Bowel Syndrome. Used in soaps and cosmetics

Half-life: N/A

Clinically important, potentially hazardous interactions with: aspirin, chlorpromazine, fluphenazine, phenothiazine, thioridazine, warfarin

Reactions

Skin	Other
Adverse effects (sic) [1]	Seizures

Note: The Medicines Control Agency (MCA) has withdrawn licenses for prescription evening primrose drug products under the brand names of Epogam and Efamast. This was because there is not enough evidence that they are effective

FAMOTIDINE

Trade name: Pepcid (Merck)

Other common trade names: *Amfamox; Apo-Famotidine; Durater; Famodil; Famoxal; Ganor; Gastro; Motiax; Mylanta AR; Nu-Famotidine; Pepcidine; Pepdul; Sigafam*

Indications: Duodenal ulcer, Gastroesophageal Reflux Disease (GERD)

Category: Antihistamine H_2-blocker

Half-life: 2.5–3.5 hours

Clinically important, potentially hazardous interactions with: cefditoren, devil's claw

Reactions

Skin	
Acne (<1%)	Erythema multiforme [1]
Acute generalized exanthematous pustulosis (AGEP) [1]	Exanthems
	Facial edema
Allergic reactions (sic) (<1%)	Pruritus (<1%) [2]
Angioedema (#<1%) [1]	Purpura [1]
Candidiasis [1]	Rash (sic) [2]
Dermatitis [2]	Side effects (sic) [1]
Dermographism [1]	Toxic epidermal necrolysis [1]
	Urticaria (<1%) [2]

Vasculitis [2]
Xerosis (<1%)

Hair
Hair – alopecia

Eyes
Periorbital edema

Cardiovascular
Flushing [1]

Other
Dysgeusia

Gynecomastia
Headache [1]
Hiccups [1]
Injection-site pain
Myalgia
Oral lesions [1]
Paresthesias (<1%) [2]
Seizures [1]
Tinnitus
Xerostomia [1]

FELBAMATE

Trade name: Felbatol (MedPointe)
Other common trade names: *Felbamyl; Taloxa*
Indications: Partial seizures
Category: Antiepileptic
Half-life: 13–23 hours

Reactions

Skin
Acne (3.4%)
Anticonvulsant hypersensitivity syndrome
 [1]
Bullous eruption (<1%)
Diaphoresis
Edema
Facial edema (3.4%)
Idiosyncratic drug reactions [1]
Lichen planus
Livedo reticularis
Lupus erythematosus
Photosensitivity (<0.01%)
Pruritus (>1%)
Purpura
Pustules [1]
Rash (sic) (3.5%)
Stevens–Johnson syndrome [1]
Toxic epidermal necrolysis [1]
Urticaria (<1%)

Hair
Hair – alopecia

Cardiovascular
Flushing
QT prolongation [1]

Other
Anaphylactoid reactions (<0.01%)
Dysgeusia (6.1%)
Foetor ex ore (halitosis)
Gingivitis
Glossitis
Headache
Myalgia (2.6%)
Oral edema (>1%)
Paresthesias (3.5%)
Thrombophlebitis
Xerostomia (2.6%)

FENOPROFEN

Trade name: Nalfon (Ranbaxy)
Other common trade names: *Fenoprex; Fenopron; Fepron; Feprona; Nalgesic; Progesic*
Indications: Arthritis
Category: Nonsteroidal anti-inflammatory (NSAID)
Half-life: 2.5–3 hours
Clinically important, potentially hazardous interactions with: methotrexate

Reactions

Skin
Acne [1]
Angioedema (<1%)
Bruising (<1%)
Bullous eruption
Diaphoresis (<0.5%)
Erythema multiforme (<1%) [1]
Exanthems [2]
Exfoliative dermatitis (<1%)
Peripheral edema (<1%)
Pruritus (3–9%) [3]
Purpura (<1%) [2]
Rash (sic) (>10%)
Stevens–Johnson syndrome (<1%)
Toxic epidermal necrolysis (<1%) [1]
Urticaria (1–3%) [2]
Vesiculobullous eruption [1]

Hair
Hair – alopecia (<1%)

Cardiovascular
Hot flashes (<1%)

Other
Anaphylactoid reactions
Aphthous stomatitis (<1%)
Dysgeusia (<1%) (metallic taste)
Glossopyrosis (<1%)
Headache
Mastodynia (<1%)
Oral ulceration
Stomatitis
Tinnitus
Xerostomia (>1%)

FENTANYL

Trade names: Actiq (Cephalon); Duragesic (Janssen)
Other common trade names: *Beatryl; Durogesic; Fentanest; Leptanal; Sublimaze*
Indications: Chronic pain
Category: Narcotic agonist analgesic
Half-life: 1.5–6 hours
Clinically important, potentially hazardous interactions with: amiodarone, amprenavir, atazanavir, cimetidine, indinavir, itraconazole, nelfinavir, ranitidine, ritonavir, saquinavir

Reactions

Skin
Clammy skin (<1%)
Diaphoresis (>10%) [3]
Edema [1]

Erythema (at application site) (<1%) [2]
Exanthems
Exfoliative dermatitis
Fixed eruption [1]

Papulo-nodular lesions (>1%)
Pruritus (3–44%) [21]
Purpura [1]
Pustules (<1%)
Rash (sic) (>1%) [2]
Urticaria (<1%)

Cardiovascular
Bradycardia [1]
Flushing (3–10%)
Hypotension [1]

Other
Anaphylactoid reactions [4]
Cough [2]
Death [3]
Dizziness [1]
Dysesthesia (<1%)
Dysgeusia (<1%)
Headache
Paresthesias (<1%)
Xerostomia (>10%) [2]

FEVERFEW

Scientific names: *Chrysanthemum parthenium; Pyrethrum parthenium; Tanacetum parthenium*
Family: Asteraceae; Compositae
Trade and other common names: Atamisa; Featerfoiul; Featherfew; Featherfoil; MIG-99; Santa Maria
Category: Stimulant and tonic
Purported indications and other uses: Fever, headache, migraine, menstrual irregularities, arthritis, psoriasis, allergy, asthma, tinnitus, vertigo, nausea, cold, earache, orthopedic disorders, swollen feet, diarrhea, dyspepsia
Half-life: N/A
Clinically important, potentially hazardous interactions with: anticoagulants, NSAIDs, warfarin

Reactions

Skin
Adverse effects (sic) (mild) [1]
Allergic reactions (sic) [1]
Angioedema (lips) [2]
Dermatitis [2]
Prurigo nodularis [1]

Other
Ageusia [2]
Bleeding [1]
Oral ulceration [2]

FLAVOXATE

Trade name: Urispas (Ortho-McNeil)
Other common trade names: *Bladderon; Genurin; Harnin; Patricin; Spasuret; Urispadol; Uronid*
Indications: Dysuria, urgency, nocturia
Category: Urinary antispasmodic
Half-life: Onset of action: 55–60 minutes
Clinically important, potentially hazardous interactions with: anticholinergics, arbutamine

---

Reactions

Skin
  Exanthems
  Rash (sic) (<1%) [1]
  Urticaria

Other
  Headache
  Hypersensitivity [1]
  Oral ulceration [1]
  Xerostomia (>10%)

FLUOXYMESTERONE

Trade names: Android-F; Halotestin (Pfizer)
Other common trade names: *Stenox; Vewon*
Indications: Breast carcinoma, hypogonadism, anemia
Category: Androgen; Antianemic; Antineoplastic
Half-life: 9.2 hours
Clinically important, potentially hazardous interactions with: anticoagulants, cyclosporine, warfarin

---

Reactions

Skin
  Acne (>10%) [12]
  Dermatitis [1]
  Edema (>10%)
  Exanthems
  Furunculosis [1]
  Lichenoid eruption [1]
  Lupus erythematosus [1]
  Pruritus
  Psoriasis [1]
  Purpura
  Seborrhea
  Seborrheic dermatitis [1]
  Striae [1]
  Urticaria

Hair
  Hair – alopecia [2]
  Hair – hirsutism (1–10%) [9]

Cardiovascular
  Flushing (1–5%) [1]

Other
  Anaphylactoid reactions
  Gynecomastia (<1%)
  Hypersensitivity (<1%)
  Injection-site pain
  Mastodynia (>10%)
  Paresthesias
  Priapism (>10%)
  Stomatitis

FLURBIPROFEN

Trade name: Ansaid (Pfizer)
Other common trade names: *Apo-Flurbiprofen; Cebutid; Flurofen; Flurozin; Froben; Lapole; Nu-Flurprofen*
Indications: Arthritis
Category: Nonsteroidal anti-inflammatory (NSAID)
Half-life: 3–4 hours
Clinically important, potentially hazardous interactions with: methotrexate

Reactions

Skin
  Angioedema (<1%) [1]
  Dermatitis [1]
  Dermatitis herpetiformis [1]
  Diaphoresis
  Discoloration
  Eczema (3–9%)
  Edema (3–9%)
  Erythema multiforme (<1%)
  Exanthems [3]
  Exfoliative dermatitis (<1%)
  Fixed eruption [1]
  Furunculosis
  Herpes simplex
  Herpes zoster
  Peripheral edema
  Photosensitivity (<1%)
  Pruritus (1–5%) [1]
  Pseudoreactions (sic) [1]
  Purpura
  Rash (sic) (1–3%)
  Seborrhea
  Side effects (sic) (6%) [2]
  Stevens–Johnson syndrome (<1%)
  Toxic epidermal necrolysis (<1%) [1]
  Ulcerations
  Urticaria (<1%)
  Vasculitis [1]

  Xerosis

Hair
  Hair – alopecia (<1%)

Nails
  Nails – changes (sic) (<1%)
  Nails – pigmentation

Eyes
  Ocular burning
  Ocular stinging

Cardiovascular
  Flushing
  Hot flashes (<1%)

Other
  Anaphylactoid reactions (<1%)
  Aphthous stomatitis
  Dysgeusia (<1%)
  Headache
  Hypersensitivity [1]
  Oral lichenoid eruption [2]
  Paresthesias (<1%)
  Parosmia (<1%)
  Stomatitis
  Tinnitus
  Vaginitis
  Xerostomia (<1%)

FOSPHENYTOIN

Trade name: Cerebyx (Eisai)
Indications: Seizure prophylaxis, status epilepticus
Category: Anticonvulsant
Half-life: 15 minutes
Clinically important, potentially hazardous interactions with: chloramphenicol, cyclosporine, disulfiram, dopamine, imatinib, itraconazole

Fosphenytoin is a prodrug of phenytoin

Reactions

Skin
  Acne (<1%)
  Bullous eruption [1]
  Chills
  Erythema multiforme (<1%) [1]
  Exanthems
  Exfoliative dermatitis (<1%) [1]
  Facial edema
  Lupus erythematosus [1]   •
  Pruritus (48.9%) [4]
  Rash (sic) (<1%)
  Stevens–Johnson syndrome
  Toxic epidermal necrolysis

Hematopoietic
  Ecchymoses

Other
  Application-site pain [1]
  Dysgeusia (3.3%)
  Gingival hypertrophy [1]
  Headache
  Hyperesthesia (2.2%)
  Paresthesias (4.4%) [2]
  Tongue disorder (sic)
  Xerostomia (4.4%)

FROVATRIPTAN

Trade name: Frova (Vernalis)
Indications: Migraine headaches
Category: 5-HT1 (serotonin) receptor agonist; Antimigraine
Half-life: 26 hours

Reactions

Skin
  Bullous eruption (<1%)
  Cheilitis (<1%)
  Diaphoresis (1%)
  Pruritus (<1%)
  Purpura (<1%)
  Rash (sic)

Eyes
  Conjunctivitis (<1%)

Cardiovascular
  Flushing (4%)
  Hot flashes (<1%)

Other
  Arthralgia (<1%)
  Bone or joint pain (3%)
  Depression (<1%)
  Dysesthesia (1%)
  Dysgeusia (<1%)

Headache
Hyperesthesia (<1%)
Myalgia (<1%)
Pain (1%)
Paresthesias (4%) [1]
Sialopenia (3%)

Sialorrhea (<1%)
Stomatitis (<1%)
Tinnitus (1%)
Toothache (1%)
Tremor (<1%)
Xerostomia

GABAPENTIN

Trade name: Neurontin (Pfizer)
Indications: Seizures
Category: Anticonvulsant
Half-life: 5–6 hours

Reactions

Skin
Acne (>1%)
Acute febrile neutrophilic dermatosis
  (Sweet's syndrome) [2]
Anticonvulsant hypersensitivity syndrome
  [1]
Bullous pemphigoid [1]
Edema [3]
Exanthems [2]
Facial edema (<1%)
Peripheral edema (1.7%) [2]
Pruritus (1.3%)
Purpura (<1%) [1]
Rash (sic) (>1%)
Stevens–Johnson syndrome [1]
Urticaria
Vasculitis

Hair
Hair – alopecia [1]

Other
Ataxia [1]
Dizziness [3]
Foetor ex ore (halitosis) [1]
Gingivitis (<1%)
Glossitis
Gynecomastia [1]
Myalgia (2%)
Myoclonus [1]
Paresthesias (<1%)
Priapism [1]
Sialorrhea
Stomatitis
Tinnitus
Tooth pigmentation
Tremor (1–10%) [1]
Xerostomia (1.7%)

GARLIC

Scientific name: *Allium sativum*
Family: Liliaceae
Trade and other common names: Ail; Ajo; Camphor of the Poor; Nectar of the Gods; Poor Man's Treacle; Rust Treacle; Stinking Rose
Category: Antioxidant; Antiseptic; Immune stimulant
Purported indications and other uses: Hypertension, hypercholesterolemia, atherosclerosis, earache, menstrual disorders, allergy, 'flu, arthritis, diarrhea, bacterial and fungal infections, tinea corporis, tinea pedis, onychomycosis, vaginitis
Half-life: N/A
Clinically important, potentially hazardous interactions with: atazanavir, chlorpropamide, hiv medications, lisinopril, olmesartan, saquinavir, ticlopidine, warfarin

Reactions

Skin
Allergic reactions (sic) [3]
Bullous eruption [1]
Burning [6]
Dermatitis [19]
Hemorrhage [1]
Pemphigus [1]
Urticaria [1]

Eyes
Rhinoconjunctivitis [1]

Other
Anaphylactoid reactions [1]
Bleeding [2]
Foetor ex ore (halitosis)
Hypersensitivity [2]
Sensitization [1]
Stomatodynia

GINGER

Scientific name: *Zingiber officinale*
Family: Zingiberaceae
Trade and other common names: African Ginger; Cochin Ginger; Gingembre; Jamaica Ginger; Race Ginger
Category: Anti-infective; Anti-nausea
Purported indications and other uses: Colic, dyspepsia, flatulence, rheumatoid arthritis, loss of appetite, nausea, vomiting, upper respiratory infections, cough, bronchitis, burns, tinnitus, flavoring agent, fragrance component
Half-life: N/A
Clinically important, potentially hazardous interactions with: heparin, ticlopidine, warfarin

Reactions

Skin
Dermatitis [1]

Other
Bleeding [1]

GINKGO BILOBA

Scientific name: *Ginkgo biloba (Mericon)*
Family: Ginkgoaceae
Trade and other common names: Fossil Tree; Japanese Silver Apricot; Maidenhair Tree; Salisburia; Tanakan; Tebonin
Category: Antidementia; Improved cognition
Purported indications and other uses: Dementia, memory loss, headache, tinnitus, dizziness, mood disturbances, hearing disorders, intermittent claudication, attention deficit hyperactivity disorder, premenstrual syndrome, heart disease
Half-life: N/A
Clinically important, potentially hazardous interactions with: anticoagulants, aspirin, diuretics, NSAIDs, phenytoin, platelet inhibitors, SSRIs, st john's wort, thiazide diuretics, trazodone, warfarin

Reactions

Skin
  Adverse effects (sic) [3]
  Allergic reactions (sic)
  Dermatitis [2]
  Erythema
  Exanthems [1]
  Pruritus
  Rash (sic)
  Vasculitis
  Vesiculation

Eyes
  Hyphema [1]

Other
  Phlebitis
  Rectal burning
  Seizures [4]
  Spontaneous bleeding [12]
  Stomatitis

Note: *Ginkgo biloba* is the oldest living tree species in the world. Ginkgo is the most frequently prescribed herbal medicine in Germany

GLATIRAMER*

Trade name: Copaxone (Teva)
Indications: Multiple sclerosis
Category: Immunosuppressive
Half-life: N/A

*****Note:** Also known as Copolymer-1

Reactions

Skin
  Acne (>2%)
  Allergic reactions (sic)
  Angioedema
  Atrophy
  Cellulitis
  Chills (4%)
  Cyst (2%)
  Dermatitis
  Diaphoresis (15%)

Eczema
Edema (3%)
Erythema (4%)
Erythema nodosum
Exanthems
Facial edema (6%)
Flu-like syndrome (26%) [1]
Fungal dermatitis
Furunculosis
Herpes simplex (4%)
Herpes zoster
Infections (50%)
Lupus erythematosus
Nodular eruption (2%)
Peripheral edema (7%)
Photosensitivity
Pigmentation
Pruritus (185)
Psoriasis
Purpura
Pustules
Rash (sic) (18%)
Striae
Urticaria
Vesiculobullous eruption
Xanthomas
Xerosis

Hair
Hair – alopecia (>2%)

Nails
Nails – changes (>2%)

Eyes
Xerophthalmia

Hematopoietic
Ecchymoses (8%)
Injection-site ecchymoses (>2%)

Cardiovascular
Flushing [1]

Other
Ageusia
Anaphylactoid reactions
Arthralgia (24%)

Bone or joint pain
Cough (>2%)
Depression (>2%)
Dizziness (>2%)
Dysgeusia (>2%)
Embolia cutis medicamentosa (Nicolau
  syndrome) [1]
Facial numbness
Gingival hemorrhage
Glossodynia
Gynecomastia
Hallucinations
Headache
Hyperesthesia (>2%)
Injection-site abscess
Injection-site atrophy
Injection-site edema
Injection-site erythema (66%) [1]
Injection-site fibrosis
Injection-site hematoma
Injection-site hemorrhage (5%)
Injection-site hypersensitivity
Injection-site induration (13%) [1]
Injection-site inflammation (49%) [1]
Injection-site lipoatrophy [1]
Injection-site pain (73%)
Injection-site pigmentation
Injection-site pruritus (40%)
Injection-site reactions (6–67%) [3]
Injection-site urticaria (5%)
Lipoatrophy [2]
Lipomatosis
Lymphedema
Mastodynia (>2%)
Moon face
Myalgia (>2%)
Myasthenia (>2%)
Myasthenia gravis [1]
Oral candidiasis
Oral ulceration
Oral vesiculation (6%)
Pain (28%)
Paresthesias (>2%)
Pharyngitis (>2%)

Priapism
Serum sickness
Sinusitis (>2%)
Stomatitis
Tenosynovitis
Tinnitus (>2%)
Tongue edema

Tongue pigmentation
Trembling
Tremor (7%)
Tumors
Ulcerative stomatitis
Vaginitis
Xerostomia (>2%)

GLUCOSAMINE

Trade names: Arthro-Aid (NutraSense); Chitosamine; Glucosamine sulfate (Rottapharm)
Other common trade names: *2-amino-2-deoxyglucose hydrochloride;; 2-amino-deoxyglucose sulfate; N-acetyl-glucosamine (NAG)*
Indications: Arthritis, osteoarthritis, cartilage repair and maintenance, strained joints, improving joint function and range of motion, alleviating joint pain
Category: Chondroprotective agent; Dietary supplement; Immunosuppressant; Nutraceutical
Half-life: N/A

Reactions

Skin
  Adverse effects (sic) (6%) [3]
  Allergic reactions (sic) (4%) [1]
  Eczema [1]
  Pruritus [1]

Cardiovascular
  Flushing [1]

Other
  Depression (6%) [1]
  Fatigue (9%) [2]
  Hypersensitivity [1]
  Oral vesiculation (7%) [1]

GLYCOPYRROLATE

Trade name: Robinul (First Horizon)
Other common trade names: *Gastrodyn; Sroton; Strodin*
Indications: Duodenal ulcer, irritable bowel syndrome
Category: Anticholinergic; Antispasmodic
Half-life: N/A
Clinically important, potentially hazardous interactions with: anticholinergics, arbutamine

Reactions

Skin
  Allergic reactions (sic)
  Hypohidrosis (>10%)
  Photosensitivity (1–10%)
  Rash (sic) (<1%)

  Urticaria
  Xerosis (>10%)

Cardiovascular
  Flushing

Other
Anhidrosis
Dysgeusia

Headache
Injection-site irritation (>10%)
Xerostomia (>10%) [2]

GOLD and GOLD COMPOUNDS

Generic names:
Auranofin
Trade name: Ridaura (GSK)
Aurothioglucose
Trade name: Solganal (Schering)

Gold sodium thiomalate (sodium aurothiomalate)
Trade name: Myochrysine (Merck)

Other common trade names: Aureotan; Aurolate; Aurothio; Miocrin; Myocrisine; Shiosol; Tauredon
Indications: Rheumatoid arthritis
Category: Antiarthritic
Half-life: 5 days

Reactions

Skin
Acne [2]
Angioedema (<1%) [1]
Angiofibromatosis [1]
Bullous eruption [3]
Bullous pemphigoid [1]
Cheilitis [2]
Chrysiasis (blue-green pigmentation) [1]
Dermatitis [59]
Eczema [3]
Erythema annulare centrifugum [1]
Erythema multiforme [2]
Erythema nodosum [4]
Exanthems (>5%) [9]
Exfoliative dermatitis [9]
Fixed eruption
Graft-versus-host reaction [1]
Granuloma annulare [2]
Herpes zoster [2]
Lichen planus (<32%) [10]
Lichen spinulosus [1]
Lichenoid eruption [8]
Lupus erythematosus [3]
Lymphocytoma cutis [1]
Lymphomatoid eosinophilic reaction [1]
Pemphigus [1]

Photosensitivity [2]
Pigmentation [19]
Pityriasis rosea [9]
Pruritus (<84%) [8]
Psoriasis [1]
Purpura [3]
Pyoderma gangrenosum
Radiation keratosis [1]
Rash (sic) (>10%) [7]
Seborrheic dermatitis [3]
Squamous cell carcinoma [2]
Toxic dermatitis [1]
Toxic epidermal necrolysis [4]
Toxicoderma [1]
Urticaria (1–10%) [7]
Vasculitis [4]
Vitiligo [1]
Xerosis [1]

Hair
Hair – alopecia (1–10%) [5]
Hair – pigmentation [1]

Nails
Nails – dystrophy [1]
Nails – exfoliation [1]
Nails – lichen planus [1]

Nails – loss [1]
Nails – onycholysis [1]
Nails – pigmentation [3]

Hematopoietic
Pancytopenia [1]

Other
Acute intermittent porphyria
Anaphylactoid reactions
Aphthous stomatitis [3]
Burning mouth syndrome [1]
Death [1]
Dysgeusia [4]
Gingivitis (>10%) [2]

Gingivostomatitis [1]
Glossitis (>10%) [2]
Headache
Hypersensitivity [1]
Injection-site pain [1]
Mucocutaneous reactions [2]
Oral lichen planus [3]
Oral lichenoid eruption [1]
Oral mucosal eruption [1]
Oral pigmentation [2]
Oral ulceration [6]
Pseudolymphoma [3]
Stomatitis (>10%) [17]
Vaginitis [1]

Note: Adverse reactions can occur months after therapy has been discontinued

GOSERELIN

Trade name: Zoladex (AstraZeneca)
Other common trade name: *Prozoladex*
Indications: Breast and prostate carcinoma, endometriosis
Category: Gonadotropin-releasing analog hormone
Half-life: 5 hours

Reactions

Skin
Chills
Diaphoresis (1–10%)
Edema (1–10%)
Rash (sic) (1–10%)
Urticaria

Hair
Hair – alopecia [1]

Cardiovascular
Hot flashes (>10%) [2]

Other
Anaphylactoid reactions [1]
Gynecomastia (>10%)
Hypersensitivity [1]
Injection-site pain (1–10%)
Injection-site papules & nodules [1]
Mastodynia (1–10%) [1]
Relapsing polychondritis [1]

GRANISETRON

Trade name: Kytril (Roche)
Other common trade name: *Kevatril*
Indications: Chemotherapy-related emesis
Category: 5-HT(3)-receptor antagonist; Antiemetic; Serotonin antagonist
Half-life: 3–4 hours; cancer patients: 10–12 hours

Reactions

Skin
  Allergic reactions (sic) [1]
  Exanthems
  Rash (sic)
  Urticaria

Hair
  Hair – alopecia (3%)

Cardiovascular
  Hot flashes (<1%)

QT prolongation [1]

Other
  Anaphylactoid reactions
  Asthenia [1]
  Dysgeusia (2%)
  Headache
  Hypersensitivity

GREEN TEA

Scientific names: *Camellia sinensis; Camellia thea; Camellia theifera; Thea bohea; Thea sinensis; Thea viridis*
Family: Theaceae
Trade and other common names: Chinese tea
Category: Astringent; Improved cognition
Purported indications and other uses: improving cognitive performance, stomach disorders, nausea, vomiting, diarrhea, anticancer, headaches, Crohn's disease. Topical: soothe sunburn, bleeding gums, reduce sweating
Half-life: N/A
Clinically important, potentially hazardous interactions with: warfarin

Note: Tea is consumed as a beverage

Reactions

None

GUARANA*

Scientific names: *Paullinia cupana; Paullinia sorbilis*
Family: Sapindaceae
Trade and other common names: Brazilian Cocoa; Cupana; Uabano; Uaranzeiro; Zoom
Category: Adaptogen; Stimulant; Tonic
Purported indications and other uses: Aphrodisiac, diarrhea, fatigue, fever, heart problems, headache, mental alertness, neuralgia, weight loss. Cosmetic products, anti-cellulite creams, shampoo for hair loss. Flavoring
Half-life: N/A
Clinically important, potentially hazardous interactions with: caffeine, clozapine, **ephedra**, ephedrine, lithium, MAO inhibitors, phenylpropanolamine, warfarin

*Note: The main constituent of Guarana is caffeine. It contains more than twice as much caffeine as coffee or tea. Excessive consumption of caffeine is contraindicated for persons with high blood pressure, cardiac disorders, diabetes, ulcers, and epilepsy

Reactions

Other
  Abdominal pain
  Adverse effects (sic) [5]
  Death [1]
  Dizziness

Insomnia
Seizures [2]
Tinnitus
Tooth pigmentation [1]

HAWTHORN (FRUIT, LEAF, FLOWER EXTRACT)

Scientific names: *Crataegus laevigata; Crataegus monogyna; Crataegus oxyacantha; Crataegus pentagyna*

Family: Rosaceae

Trade and other common names: Arterio-K; Aubepine; Basticrat; Born; Cardiplant; Cordapur; Coronal; Cratamed; Harthorne; Haw; HeartCare (Nature's Way); Hedgethorne; Maythorn; Nan Shanzha; Naranocor; Regulacor; Shanzha; Thorn Plum; Whitethorn

Category: Improves cardiac function

Purported indications and other uses: Amenorrhea, arrhythmias, atherosclerosis, diuretic, hyperlipidemia, hypertension, hypotension, sedative, appetite stimulant, arthritis, enteritis, indigestion, sore throats. **Topical:** boils, sores and ulcers

Half-life: N/A

Clinically important, potentially hazardous interactions with: digoxin, vasodilators

Note: The American Herbal Products Association (AHPA) gives hawthorn a class 1 safety rating, indicating that it is very safe. However, hawthorn should be used with caution in patients with heart disease

---

Reactions

Skin
  Allergic reactions (sic)
  Diaphoresis [1]
  Rash (sic) (hands) [2]
  Toxicoderma [1]

Other
  Dizziness [2]
  Hypersensitivity [1]

HENNA*

Scientific names: *Lawsonia alba; Lawsonia inermis*

Family: Lythraceae

Trade and other common names: Alcanna; Egyptian Privet; Hinai; Hinna; Inai; Jamaica Kina; Lawsone (2-hydroxy-1:4naphthaquione); Mehandi; Mehndi

Category: Anti-inflammatory

Purported indications and other uses: Analgesic, antipyretic, seborrheic dermatitis, fungal infections, gastrointestinal ulcers, sunscreen, dandruff, scabies, headache, jaundice, decorative tattoos, Used in cosmetics, body paint, hair dyes, hair care products

Half-life: N/A

Note: Black Henna is Henna plus paraphenylenediamine (PPD). PPD is added to henna to make it stain black. PPD is a transdermal toxin and may be used alone as hair dye or to stain skin black. Other products called 'black henna' may have indigo or food dyes added, and are generally not harmful to the skin

Reactions

Skin
 Adverse effects (sic) [2]
 Allergic reactions (sic) [3]
 Bullous eruption
 Burning
 Dermatitis [31]
 Eczema [1]
 Edema [3]
 Erythema [3]
 Erythema multiforme [1]
 Keloid [1]
 Lichenoid eruption [4]

Photosensitivity
 Pigmentation [3]
 Pruritus [3]
 Psoriasis [1]
 Rash (sic)
 Sensitivity [1]
 Urticaria [2]

Other
 Death [3]
 Hypersensitivity [10]
 Side effects (sic) [1]

Note: Adverse side effects to pure henna are rare; those reported above may be due to additives. Henna tattoos were popularized by Madonna. Her black patterns, however, were created with body paint, not henna

HORSE CHESTNUT (BARK, FLOWER, LEAF, SEED)

Scientific name: *Aesculus hippocastanum*
Family: Hippocastanaceae
Trade and other common names: Buckeye; Hippocastani; Marron Europeen; Venostat; Venostatin Retard
Category: Diuretic
Purported indications and other uses: Oral: malaria, dysentery, tinnitus, pancreatitis, cough, arthritis, rheumatism, chronic venous insufficiency. **Topical:** lupus, skin ulcers eczema, phlebitis, varicose veins, hemorrhoids, rectal problems
Half-life: N/A
Clinically important, potentially hazardous interactions with: heparin, NSAIDs, ticlopidine, warfarin

Reactions

Skin
 Adverse effects (sic) (mild) [1]
 Dermatitis (flower) [1]
 Purpura [1]

Other
 Anaphylactoid reactions (seed) [1]
 Depression (seed)
 Twitching (seed)

*Note: The active ingredient is a toxic glycoside, escin

HYALURONIC ACID

Synonyms: Hyaluronidase; Hyaluronan; Hyaluran; Hyaluronate sodium
Trade names: Adant; ARTZ; BioHy; DermaDeep; DermaLive; Hyalgan; Hylaform; Hylan G-F 20 (Synvisc); Juvederm; Orthovisc; Perlane (Q-Med AB); Restylane Fine Lines (Medicis); Supartz
Indications: Oral: joint disorders. **Injection:** adjunct in eye surgery, viscosupplementation in orthopedics, cosmetic surgery. **Topical:** wounds, burns, skin ulcers, stomatitis
Category: Glycoaminoglycan; Immune modulator
Half-life: 2.5–5.5 minutes
Clinically important, potentially hazardous interactions with: NSAIDs, oral anticoagulants

Reactions

Skin

Acne (0.1–29%) [1]
Adverse effects (sic) [9]
Dermatitis (24%) [1]
Erythema multiforme [1]
Granulomas [9]
Herpes simplex
Infections [2]
Inflammation [3]
Irritation [1]
Upper respiratory infection

Other

Anaphylactoid reactions [1]
Arthralgia [6]
Back pain
Bronchitis

Chondritis (<11%) [2]
Depression
Gouty tophi [3]
Headache
Hypersensitivity [1]
Injection-site bruising
Injection-site edema (0.1–20%) [7]
Injection-site erythema (0.1–47%) [3]
Injection-site nodules [2]
Injection-site pain (8–47%) [11]
Injection-site pruritus
Injection-site reactions (sic) (<11%) [9]
Pneumonia
Sinusitis
Systemic reactions [1]
Tooth disorder

Note: Most reported reactions relate to orthopedic use

HYDROCODONE*

Trade names: Bacomine; Ban-Tuss HC; Codamine; Duratuss (UCB Pharma); Entex HC (Andrx); Hycotuss (Endo); Lortab (UCB Pharma); Maxidone (Watson); Morcomine; Norco (Watson); Prolex-DH; Propachem; Ru-Tuss; Tussgen; Tussionex (Celltech); Tussogest; Vicodin (Abbott); Vicoprofen (Abbott); Zydone (Endo)
Indications: Acute pain, coughing
Category: Narcotic analgesic antitussive
Half-life: 3.8 hours

Reactions

Skin
  Diaphoresis
  Edema
  Erythema multiforme
  Exanthems [1]
  Pruritus (1–10%) [3]
  Rash (sic) (>10%)
  Stevens–Johnson syndrome

  Toxic epidermal necrolysis
  Urticaria (>10%)

Cardiovascular
  Flushing
  Hot flashes

Other
  Headache
  Xerostomia

*Note: Hydrocodone is included in many combination drugs. Other medications that can be included in these preparations include: phenylpropanolamine, phenylephrine, pyrilamine, pseudoephedrine, acetaminophen, ibuprofen, and others

HYDROMORPHONE

Trade name: Dilaudid (Abbott)
Other common trade names: *Dilaudid HP; HydroStat IR; Palladone*
Indications: Pain
Category: Narcotic analgesic antitussive
Half-life: 1–3 hours
Clinically important, potentially hazardous interactions with: cimetidine

Reactions

Skin
  Diaphoresis
  Exanthems [1]
  Pruritus (1–11%) [1]
  Rash (sic) (<1%)
  Urticaria (<1%)

Hair
  Hair – alopecia

Cardiovascular
  Flushing (1–10%)

Other
  Dizziness [1]
  Dysgeusia
  Injection-site reactions (sic)
  Paresthesias
  Xerostomia (1–10%)

HYDROXYCHLOROQUINE

Trade name: Plaquenil (Sanofi-Aventis)
Other common trade names: *Ercoquin; Oxiklorin; Plaquinol; Quensyl; Toremonil; Yuma*
Indications: Malaria, lupus erythematosus, rheumatoid arthritis
Category: Antimalarial; Antirheumatic
Half-life: elimination in blood: 50 days
Clinically important, potentially hazardous interactions with: chloroquine, cholestyramine, dapsone, penicillamine

Reactions

Skin
Acute generalized exanthematous pustulosis (AGEP) [4]
Angioedema (<1%)
Atrophy [1]
Bullous eruption [2]
Dermatitis [1]
Dermatomyositis [1]
Erythema annulare centrifugum [3]
Erythema multiforme (<1%) [1]
Erythema nodosum [1]
Erythroderma [2]
Exanthems (1–5%) [4]
Exfoliative dermatitis [4]
Fixed eruption (<1%)
Lichenoid eruption [4]
Photosensitivity [7]
Phototoxicity [1]
Pigmentation (1–10%) [6]
Pruritus (>10%) [13]
Psoriasis (exacerbation) [10]
Purpura
Pustular psoriasis [3]
Pustules [1]
Rash (sic) (1–10%) [1]
Stevens–Johnson syndrome [1]
Telangiectasia [1]
Toxic epidermal necrolysis [2]

Urticaria [3]
Vasculitis [1]

Hair
Hair – alopecia
Hair – pigmentation (bleaching) (1–10%) [7]

Nails
Nails – discoloration [1]
Nails – pigmentation [3]

Eyes
Ocular toxicity [1]

Other
Death [1]
Dysgeusia [2]
Gingival pigmentation [1]
Headache
Lymphoproliferative disease [1]
Mucosal atrophy [1]
Myalgia [2]
Oral pigmentation [5]
Oral ulceration
Porphyria [7]
Stomatitis [1]
Stomatopyrosis
Tinnitus

HYDROXYUREA

Trade names: Droxia (Bristol-Myers Squibb); Hydrea (Bristol-Myers Squibb); Mylocel
Other common trade names: *Litalir; Onco-Carbide*
Indications: Leukemia, malignant tumors
Category: Antineoplastic
Half-life: 3–4 hours
Clinically important, potentially hazardous interactions with: adefovir, aldesleukin

Reactions

Skin
Acral erythema [6]
Acral ulcers [1]
Acrodermatitis perstans [1]
Acute febrile neutrophilic dermatosis (Sweet's syndrome) [1]
Atrophy [1]
Baboon syndrome [1]
Collodion-like skin [1]
Dermatitis (dry, scaly) [2]
Dermatomyositis [16]
Erythema gyratum [1]
Erythema multiforme (<1%)
Exanthems (1–10%) [1]
Facial erythema (<1%) [1]
Fixed eruption (<1%) [4]
Ichthyosis [2]
Infections [1]
Keratoacanthoma [1]
Keratoses [2]
Lichen planus [3]
Lichenoid acrodermatitis [1]
Lichenoid eruption [2]
Lupus erythematosus [2]
Palmar–plantar desquamation [6]
Peripheral edema [1]
Photo-recall [2]
Photosensitivity [1]
Pigmentation (1–58%) [14]
Poikiloderma [1]
Pruritus (<1%) [3]
Psoriasis [1]
Purpura [2]
Rash (sic)

Side effects (sic) (7–35%) [3]
Squamous cell carcinoma [2]
Telangiectasia [2]
Ulceration of foot [1]
Ulcerations [23]
Ulcerations of legs (29%) [10]
Urticaria
Vasculitis [7]
Xerosis (1–10%) [6]

Hair
Hair – alopecia (1–10%) [6]

Nails
Nails – atrophic [3]
Nails – dystrophy [1]
Nails – melanonychia [1]
Nails – onycholysis [2]
Nails – pigmentation (9%) [18]

Other
Death [1]
Gangrene (toes) [1]
Glossitis [1]
Mucocutaneous eruption [1]
Myositis [1]
Oral lesions [2]
Oral pigmentation (<29%) [2]
Oral squamous cell carcinoma [1]
Oral ulceration [4]
Porphyria cutanea tarda [1]
Scleral pigmentation [1]
Stomatitis (>10%) [3]
Tongue pigmentation (<29%) [3]
Tumors [5]

HYOSCYAMINE

Synonyms: Hyoscyamine sulfate; hyoscyamine sulfate

Trade names: Anaspaz; Cytospaz; Donnamar; ED-SPAZ; Gastrosed; Hyco; Hycosol SI; Hyospaz; IB-Stat (InKline); Levbid (Schwarz); Levsin (Schwarz); Levsin/SL (Schwarz); Levsinex (Schwarz); Medispaz; Nulev (Schwarz); Pasmex; Setamine; Urised

Other common trade names: *Duboisine; Egacene Durettes; Egazil; Peptard*

Indications: Treatment of gastrointestinal tract disorders caused by spasm. Adjunctive therapy for peptic ulcers, cystitis, parkinsonism, biliary & renal colic

Category: Anticholinergic

Duration of action: 13–38 min

Clinically important, potentially hazardous interactions with: anticholinergics, arbutamine

Reactions

Skin

Allergic reactions (sic)
Hypohidrosis (>10%)
Photosensitivity (1–10%)
Rash (sic) (<1%)
Urticaria
Xerosis (>10%)

Cardiovascular

Flushing

Other

Ageusia
Anaphylactoid reactions
Dysgeusia
Headache
Injection-site inflammation (>10%)
Xerostomia (>10%)

IBUPROFEN

Trade names: Advil (Wyeth); Genpril; Haltran; Medipren; Midol 220; Motrin (McNeil); Nuprin; Pamprin; Profen; Rufen; Trendar; Vicoprofen (Abbott)

Other common trade names: *Act-3; Actiprofen; Anco; Apsifen; Brufen; Ebufac; Lidifen; Proflex; Tabalom; Urem*

Indications: Arthritis, pain

Category: Antipyretic; Nonsteroidal anti-inflammatory (NSAID)

Half-life: 2–4 hours

Clinically important, potentially hazardous interactions with: aspirin, boswellia, diuretics, methotrexate, NSAIDs, oxycodone hydrochloride, salicylates, tacrolimus, urokinase

Reactions

Skin

Angioedema (<1%) [5]
Bullous eruption (<1%) [3]
Bullous pemphigoid [2]
Dermatitis (<1%) [3]

Dermatitis herpetiformis [1]
Diaphoresis [1]
Eczema [1]
Edema (<1%)
Erythema multiforme (<1%) [7]

Erythema nodosum (1–5%) [1]
Exanthems [9]
Fixed eruption (<1%) [14]
Lichenoid eruption [1]
Linear IgA dermatosis [1]
Livedo reticularis [1]
Lupus erythematosus [5]
Pemphigus [1]
Photosensitivity [6]
Pruritus (1–5%) [5]
Psoriasis (palms) [2]
Purpura [1]
Rash (sic) (>10%) [1]
Stevens–Johnson syndrome (<1%) [2]
Toxic epidermal necrolysis (<1%) [2]
Urticaria (>10%) [9]
Vasculitis [8]
Vesiculobullous eruption [2]

Hair

Hair – alopecia (<1%) [2]
Hair – disorders [1]

Nails

Nails – changes (sic) [1]
Nails – onycholysis [1]

Eyes

Periorbital edema [1]
Visual disturbances [2]

Cardiovascular

Flushing
Hot flashes (<1%)

Other

Anaphylactoid reactions (<1%) [5]
Aphthous stomatitis
Death [1]
DRESS syndrome [1]
Embolia cutis medicamentosa (Nicolau
  syndrome) [2]
Gingival ulceration (<1%)
Gynecomastia (<1%)
Headache
Hypersensitivity [2]
Impaired wound healing [1]
Myalgia [1]
Oral lesions [1]
Oral lichenoid eruption [1]
Oral ulceration [1]
Paresthesias
Pseudolymphoma [1]
Pseudoporphyria [2]
Rhabdomyolysis [1]
Serum sickness [1]
Stomatitis
Tinnitus
Xerostomia (<1%)

INDOMETHACIN

Synonym: indometacin
Other common trade names: *Amuno; Apo-Indomethacin; Durametacin; Imbrilon; Indochron; Indolar SR; Indotec; Nu-Indo; Rhodacine; Vonum*
Indications: Arthritis
Category: Antipyretic; Nonsteroidal anti-inflammatory (NSAID)
Half-life: 4.5 hours
Clinically important, potentially hazardous interactions with: aldesleukin, aspirin, diflunisal, diuretics, methotrexate, NSAIDs, sermorelin, triamterene, urokinase

Reactions

Skin

Angioedema (<1%) [2]

Bullous eruption (<1%) [2]
Dermatitis [5]

Dermatitis herpetiformis (exacerbation) [2]
Diaphoresis (<1%)
Eczema [1]
Edema (3–9%) [1]
Erythema multiforme (<1%) [1]
Erythema nodosum (<1%) [1]
Exanthems (1–5%) [7]
Exfoliative dermatitis (<1%) [1]
Fixed eruption [2]
Generalized eruption (sic) [1]
Granulomas (plasma cell) [1]
Lichen planus [1]
Pemphigus
Peripheral edema
Petechiae (>1%)
Photosensitivity [1]
Pruritus (1–10%) [3]
Psoriasis [7]
Purpura (<1%) [5]
Pustular psoriasis [1]
Rash (sic) (>10%) [1]
Reiter's syndrome (exacerbation) [1]
Side effects (sic) [1]
Stevens–Johnson syndrome (<1%)
Toxic epidermal necrolysis (<1%) [6]
Urticaria [7]
Urticaria pigmentosa [1]
Vasculitis (<1%) [5]

Hair
Hair – alopecia (<1%)

Nails
Nails – onycholysis

Eyes
Periorbital edema [2]

Hematopoietic
Ecchymoses (<1%)

Cardiovascular
Angina [1]
Flushing (>1%)
Hot flashes (<1%)

Other
Ageusia [1]
Anaphylactoid reactions (<1%)
Aphthous stomatitis
Gynecomastia (<1%)
Headache
Hypersensitivity (<1%)
Oral lesions (<7%) [2]
Oral lichenoid eruption [1]
Oral ulceration [4]
Paresthesias (<1%)
Pseudolymphoma [1]
Pseudoporphyria [1]
Serum sickness [1]
Temporal arteritis [2]
Tinnitus
Tongue edema [1]
Ulcerative stomatitis (<1%) [1]
Xerostomia

INFLIXIMAB

Trade name: Remicade (Centocor)
Indications: Crohn's disease
Category: Monoclonal antibody; Tumor necrosis factor alpha blocker
Half-life: 9.5 days

Reactions

Skin
Acute febrile neutrophilic dermatosis
  (Sweet's syndrome) [1]
Adverse effects (sic) [1]

Allergic reactions (sic) [1]
Bullous eruption [1]
Candidiasis (5%) [1]
Cellulitis [1]

Chills (5–9%) [1]
Edema [2]
Exanthems [3]
Facial edema [1]
Folliculitis [1]
Herpes simplex [1]
Herpes zoster [1]
Infections (21%) [6]
Lichenoid eruption [1]
Lupus erythematosus [6]
Lupus syndrome [3]
Lymphoma [3]
Molluscum contagiosum (eyelids) [1]
Necrotizing fasciitis [1]
Peripheral edema [1]
Pernio [1]
Photosensitivity [1]
Pruritus (5%) [4]
Psoriasis [3]
Pustules [2]
Rash (sic) (6%) [7]
Red man syndrome [1]
Ulcerations (foot) [1]
Upper respiratory infection [1]
Urticaria [3]
Urticaria [1]
Vasculitis [3]

Hair
Hair – alopecia areata [1]

Cardiovascular
Chest pain [1]
Congestive heart failure [1]
Hypertension [1]

Other
Abdominal pain [1]
Anaphylactoid reactions [5]
Application-site reactions (<4%) (mild) [6]
Arthralgia [6]
Back pain [1]
Bronchitis [1]
Cough [1]
Death [5]
Depression [1]
Dizziness [1]
Fatigue [1]
Fever [3]
Headache [2]
Hypersensitivity [4]
Injection-site reactions (sic) (6%) [5]
Lymphadenopathy [1]
Lymphoproliferative disease [1]
Myalgia (5%) [5]
Oral mucositis [1]
Pain [1]
Paresthesias (1–4%) [1]
Parkinsonism [1]
Pharyngitis [1]
Pneumonia [2]
Polychondritis [1]
Polymyositis [2]
Rhinitis [1]
Seizures [1]
Serum sickness (<3%) [2]
Sinusitis [1]
Ulcerative stomatitis [1]

IPRATROPIUM

Trade names: Atrovent (Boehringer Ingelheim); Combivent (Boehringer Ingelheim); Duoneb (DEY)
Other common trade names: *Alti-Ipratropium; Novo-Ipramide*
Indications: Bronchospasm
Category: Anticholinergic; Antimuscarinic bronchodilator
Half-life: 2 hours

Combivent is albuterol and ipratropium

Reactions

Skin
  Dermatitis [1]
  Exanthems
  Miliaria profunda [1]
  Pruritus (<1%)
  Rash (sic) (1.2%)
  Urticaria (<1%)

Hair
  Hair – alopecia (<1%)

Cardiovascular
  Flushing (<1%)

Other
  Anaphylactoid reactions [1]
  Death [1]
  Dysgeusia (1%) (metallic taste) [2]
  Headache
  Oral lesions (1–5%) [1]
  Oral ulceration (<1%) [2]
  Paresthesias (<1%)
  Stomatitis (<1%)
  Trembling (1–10%)
  Xerostomia (3.2%) [1]

ISOFLURANE

Trade names: Forane (Baxter); Forane (Baxter)
Other common trade names: *Aerrane; Floran; Forene; Forthane; Isofluran; Isoflurano; Isofor; Isorane; Lisorane; Sofloran; Tensocold*
Indications: Maintenance of general anesthesia
Category: General inhalation anesthetic
Onset of action: 7-10 minutes
Clinically important, potentially hazardous interactions with: cisatracurium, doxacurium, muscle relaxants, pancuronium, rapacuronium

Reactions

Skin
  Shivering (post-operative)

ISOSORBIDE DINITRATE

Synonyms: ISD; ISDN
Trade names: Dilatrate-SR (Schwarz); Isordil (Wyeth); Sorbitrate (AstraZeneca)
Other common trade names: *Apo-ISDN; Cedocard; Coradur*
Indications: Angina pectoris
Category: Antianginal; Vasodilator
Half-life: 4 hours (oral)
Clinically important, potentially hazardous interactions with: sildenafil

Reactions

Skin
  Diaphoresis
  Edema (<1%) [1]
  Exanthems [1]
  Pallor
  Peripheral edema [1]

Cardiovascular
  Bradycardia [1]
  Flushing (>10%) [1]
  Hypotension [1]

Other
  Headache
  Xerostomia

ISOSORBIDE MONONITRATE

Synonym: ISMN
Trade names: Imdur (Schering); Ismo; Monoket (Schwarz)
Indications: Angina pectoris
Half-life: ~4 hours
Clinically important, potentially hazardous interactions with: sildenafil

Reactions

Skin
  Diaphoresis
  Edema (<1%)
  Peripheral edema [1]
  Pruritus (<1%)
  Rash (sic) (<1%)

Cardiovascular
  Atrial fibrillation [1]
  Flushing (>10%) [1]

Other
  Headache
  Hyperesthesia (<1%)
  Tooth disorder (sic) (<1%)

ISRADIPINE

Trade name: DynaCirc (Reliant)
Other common trade names: *Dynacirc SRO; Lomir; Lomir SRO; Prescal; Vascal*
Indications: Hypertension
Category: Antihypertensive; Calcium channel blocker
Half-life: 8 hours
Clinically important, potentially hazardous interactions with: epirubicin, imatinib, phenytoin

Reactions

Skin
  Diaphoresis (<1%)
  Edema (7.2%) [6]
  Exanthems (1.5%) [2]
  Peripheral edema
  Pruritus (<6%) [1]
  Rash (sic) (1.5%)
  Urticaria (<1%)

Cardiovascular
  Flushing (2–9%) [8]

  QT prolongation [1]
  Torsades de pointes [1]

Other
  Dizziness (9%) [1]
  Gingival hypertrophy (<1%)
  Headache (9%) [1]
  Oral lesions (6%) [1]
  Paresthesias (<1%)
  Xerostomia (<1%)

KAVA

Scientific name: *Piper methysticum*
Family: Piperaceae
Trade and other common names: Ava; Awa; Intoxicating Pepper; Kavosporal; Kew; Sakau; Tonga
Category: Anxiolytic; Sedative
Purported indications and other uses: Psychosis, depression, headache, migraines, colds, rheumatism, cystitis, vaginal prolapse, otitis, abscesses, antistress, analgesic, local anesthetic, anticonvulsant
Half-life: N/A
Clinically important, potentially hazardous interactions with: alcohol, alprazolam, benzodiazepines, escitalopram, levodopa

Note: Products containing kava have been implicated in cases of severe liver toxicity. Serious adverse effects include hepatitis, cirrhosis and liver failure. At least one patient required a liver transplant. Kava has now been banned in many countries

Reactions

Skin
  Adverse effects (sic) [6]
  Dermopathy (pellagra-like syndrome) [3]

  Lymphocytic inflammation of the dermis
  Photosensitivity
  Pigmentation (yellow)

Pruritus
Rash (sic)
Scaly dermatitis
Seborrheic dermatitis [1]
Xerosis

Hair
Hair – pigmentation

Nails
Nails – pigmentation

Other
Death [1]
Dizziness [1]
Hypersensitivity [1]
Mouth numbness
Parkinsonism [1]
Seizures [1]
Side effects (sic) [3]

Note: Kava was discovered by Captain Cook, who named the plant 'intoxicating pepper.' In the South Pacific, kava is a popular social drink, similar to alcohol in Western societies

KETOPROFEN

Trade names: Orudis (Sanofi-Aventis); Oruvail (Wyeth)
Other common trade names: *Alrheumat; Alrheumun; Aneol; Bi-Profenid; Gabrilen Retard; Keduril; Novo-Keto; Rhodis; Rhovail*
Indications: Arthritis
Category: Nonsteroidal anti-inflammatory (NSAID) analgesic
Half-life: 1.5–4 hours
Clinically important, potentially hazardous interactions with: aspirin, methotrexate, probenecid

Reactions

Skin
Allergic reactions (sic) (<1%)
Angioedema (<1%) [1]
Bullous eruption (<1%)
Dermatitis [19]
Diaphoresis (<1%) [1]
Eczema (<1%) [2]
Erythema multiforme (<1%)
Exanthems [1]
Exfoliative dermatitis (<1%)
Facial edema (<1%)
Pemphigus (localized) [1]
Peripheral edema (1–3%)
Photosensitivity [24]
Pigmentation (<1%)
Pruritus (1–10%) [1]
Psoriasis [1]
Purpura (<1%) [1]

Rash (sic) (>10%)
Side effects (sic) (<1%) [1]
Stevens–Johnson syndrome (<1%)
Toxic epidermal necrolysis (<1%) [1]
Urticaria (<1%) [1]

Hair
Hair – alopecia (<1%) [1]

Nails
Nails – onycholysis (<1%) [1]

Cardiovascular
Hot flashes (<1%)

Other
Acute intermittent porphyria
Anaphylactoid reactions (<1%) [2]
Aphthous stomatitis
Dysgeusia (<1%)
Gynecomastia (<1%)

Headache
Myalgia (<1%)
Oral lesions [1]
Oral mucosal paresthesias [1]
Paresthesias (<1%)
Pseudolymphoma [1]

Pseudoporphyria [2]
Sialorrhea (<1%)
Stomatitis (<1%)
Tinnitus
Xerostomia (<1%) [1]

KETOROLAC

Trade names: Acular (Allergan); Toradol (Roche)
Other common trade names: *Dolac; Kelac; Ketonic; Nodine; Topadol; Torolac; Torvin*
Indications: Pain
Category: Nonsteroidal anti-inflammatory (NSAID)
Half-life: 2–8 hours
Clinically important, potentially hazardous interactions with: aspirin, methotrexate, probenecid, salicylates

Reactions

Skin
Allergic reactions (sic) [1]
Angioedema [1]
Dermatitis (3–9%)
Diaphoresis (1–10%) [1]
Edema (3–9%)
Exanthems (3–9%) [1]
Excoriations [1]
Exfoliative dermatitis (<1%)
Pruritus (3–9%)
Purpura (>1%) [1]
Rash (sic) (>1%)
Side effects (sic) (0.7%) [1]
Stevens–Johnson syndrome (<1%)
Stinging (from topical) [1]
Toxic epidermal necrolysis (<1%)
Urticaria [1]

Cardiovascular
Flushing (<1%)

Other
Anaphylactoid reactions (<1%)
Aphthous stomatitis (<1%) [1]
Dizziness [1]
Dysgeusia
Headache
Hypersensitivity [1]
Injection-site lichenoid reaction [1]
Injection-site pain (1–10%)
Myalgia
Paresthesias
Stomatitis (>1%)
Tinnitus
Tongue edema (<1%)
Xerostomia [1]

L-CARNITINE

Trade names: Aplegin; L-Carnipure
Other common trade names: *Acetyl-L-carnitine; B(t)Factor; Carnitine; Carnitor; Levocarnitine; Propionyl-L-carnitine; Vitacarn; Vitamin B(t)*
Indications: Improves lipid metabolism, red blood cell count, and antioxidant status, chronic fatigue syndrome, dementia, angina, post-MI cardioprotection, congestive heart failure, valproate toxicity, anorexia
Category: Dietary supplement

Note: Mixed D, L-carnitine has been associated with myasthenic syndrome.

Reactions

None

LAMOTRIGINE

Synonyms: BW-430C; LTG
Trade name: Lamictal (GSK)
Indications: Epilepsy
Category: Anticonvulsant
Half-life: 24 hours
Clinically important, potentially hazardous interactions with: oral contraceptives

---

Reactions

Skin

Acne (1.3%)
Acute generalized exanthematous
  pustulosis (AGEP) [1]
Adverse effects (sic) [1]
Angioedema (1–10%) [1]
Anticonvulsant hypersensitivity syndrome
  [5]
Bullous eruption [1]
Diaphoresis (<1%)
Eczema (<1%)
Erythema (1–10%) [1]
Erythema multiforme [3]
Exanthems (1–10%) [12]
Facial edema (<1%)
Fixed eruption [1]
Flu-like syndrome (7%)
Hyperhidrosis [1]
Lupus erythematosus [1]

Petechiae (<1%)
Photosensitivity [2]
Pruritus (3.1%) [1]
Rash (sic) (10–20%) [24]
Stevens–Johnson syndrome (1–10%) [20]
Toxic epidermal necrolysis [26]
Urticaria (<1%)
Xerosis (<1%)

Hair

Hair – alopecia (1.3%)
Hair – hirsutism (<1%)

Hematopoietic

Ecchymoses (<1%)

Cardiovascular

Flushing (<1%)
Hot flashes (1–10%)

Other
Anaphylactoid reactions [1]
Death
Dizziness [1]
Dysgeusia (<1%) [1]
Foetor ex ore (halitosis) (<1%)
Gingival hypertrophy (<1%)
Gingivitis (<1%)
Headache [1]
Hyperesthesia (<1%)
Hypersensitivity (1–10%) [17]
Lymphadenopathy [1]

Myalgia (>1%)
Oral ulceration (<1%)
Paresthesias (>1%)
Porphyria [1]
Pseudolymphoma [1]
Sialorrhea (<1%)
Stomatitis (<1%)
Tic disorder [1]
Tremor [4]
Vaginitis (4.1%)
Vulvovaginal candidiasis (<1%)
Xerostomia (1%)

LAVENDER

Scientific names: *Lavandula angustifolia; Lavandula dentata; Lavandula spica; Lavandula vera*
Family: Lamiaceae
Trade and other common names: Alhucema; English Lavender; French Lavender; Spanish Lavender; Spike Lavender
Category: Sedative
Purported indications and other uses: Restlessness, insomnia, loss of appetite, flatulence, colic, giddiness, nervous headache, migraine, toothache, sprains, neuralgia, rheumatism, acne, pimples, nausea, vomiting. Flavoring, fragrance, insect repellent
Half-life: N/A

Reactions

Skin
Dermatitis [2]

LEFLUNOMIDE

Trade name: Arava (Sanofi-Aventis)
Indications: Rheumatoid arthritis
Category: Antimetabolite; Immunosuppressant
Half-life: 14–15 days

Reactions

Skin
Acne (1–10%)
Allergic reactions (sic) (2%) [4]
Bullous eruption [2]
Dermatitis (1–10%)
Diaphoresis (1–10%)

Eczema (2%)
Exfoliative dermatitis [1]
Herpes (1–10%)
Infections (4%) [1]
Lichenoid eruption [1]
Lupus erythematosus [1]

Nodular eruption (1–10%)
Peripheral edema (1–10%)
Pigmentation (1–10%)
Pruritus (4%) [1]
Purpura (1–10%)
Rash (sic) (10%) [9]
Squamous cell carcinoma [1]
Stevens–Johnson syndrome
Toxic epidermal necrolysis
Ulcerations (1–10%)
Urticaria (<1%)
Vasculitis (1–10%) [1]
Xerosis (2%)

Hair
Hair – alopecia (10%) [11]
Hair – alopecia areata [1]
Hair – pigmentation (1–10%)

Nails
Nails – changes (sic) (1–10%)

Other
Anaphylactoid reactions (<1%)
Death [1]
Dysgeusia (1–10%)
Gingivitis (1–10%)
Headache
Myalgia (1–10%)
Oral candidiasis (3%)
Oral ulceration (3%)
Paresthesias (2%)
Stomatitis (3%)
Tendon rupture (1–10%)
Tooth disorder (sic) (1–10%)
Vulvovaginal candidiasis (1–10%)
Xerostomia (1–10%)

LEUCOVORIN

Synonyms: citrovorum factor; folinic acid
Trade name: Leucovorin
Other common trade names: *Antrex; Citrec; Lederfolin; Refolinin; Rescufolin; Rescuvolin*
Indications: Overdose of methotrexate
Category: Antidote; Methotrexate toxicity prophylactic agent
Half-life: 15 minutes

Reactions

Skin
Erythema (<1%)
Pruritus (<1%)
Rash (sic) (<1%)
Urticaria (<1%)

Hair
Hair – alopecia [1]

Other
Anaphylactoid reactions (<1%)
Death [1]
Hypersensitivity
Mucositis [1]
Oral ulceration [1]
Phlebitis [1]

LEUPROLIDE

Synonym: leuprorelin acetate
Trade names: Eligard (Sanofi-Aventis); Lupron (TAP); Viadur (Bayer)
Other common trade names: *Carcinil; Enantone; Lucrin; Procren Depot; Procrin; Tapros*
Indications: Prostate carcinoma, endometriosis
Category: Gonadotropin-releasing hormone
Half-life: 3–4 hours

Reactions

Skin
　Acne
　Dermatitis (5%)
　Dermatitis herpetiformis [1]
　Diaphoresis
　Edema (1–10%)
　Exanthems
　Lupus erythematosus [1]
　Nodular eruption [1]
　Peripheral edema (4–12%) [1]
　Photosensitivity
　Pigmentation (<5%)
　Pruritus (<5%)
　Purpura (<1%)
　Rash (sic) (1–10%)
　Stickiness [1]
　Urticaria
　Xerosis (<5%)

Hair
　Hair – alopecia (<5%)
　Hair – hypertrichosis (<1%)

Hematopoietic
　Ecchymoses (<5%)

Cardiovascular
　Flushing (61%) [1]
　Hot flashes (12–57%) [3]

Other
　Depression [1]
　Dysgeusia (<5%)
　Gynecomastia (7%)
　Headache
　Injection-site granuloma [2]
　Injection-site inflammation (2%) [1]
　Injection-site pruritus [1]
　Injection-site reactions (24%) [1]
　Mastodynia (7%)
　Myalgia [1]
　Paresthesias (<5%)
　Thrombophlebitis (2%)
　Vaginitis

LEVETIRACETAM

Trade name: Keppra (UCB Pharma)
Indications: Partial onset seizures
Category: Anticonvulsant
Half-life: 7 hours

Reactions

Skin
　Edema [1]

　Flu-like syndrome [1]
　Fungal dermatitis (>1%)

Infections (sic) (13–26%) [5]
Rash (sic) (>1%)

Hematopoietic
Ecchymoses (<1%)

Other
Asthenia (<22%) [3]

Dizziness (9–18%) [4]
Gingivitis (>1%)
Headache (25%) [1]
Pain [1]
Paresthesias (2%)

LEVOBUPIVACAINE

Trade name: Chirocaine (Purdue)
Indications: Regional anesthesia for surgery, postoperative pain management
Category: Local anesthetic
Half-life: 1.3 hours

Reactions

Skin
Angioedema
Chills
Diaphoresis (<1%)
Edema (<1%)
Erythema
Pigmentation (<1%)
Pruritus (3.7%)
Purpura (1.4%)
Rash (sic) [1]
Shivering [1]
Urticaria

Other
Anaphylactoid reactions
Back pain (6%)
Cough (1%)
Hyperesthesia (3%)
Mastodynia (1%)
Pain (7–18%)
Paresthesias (2%)
Seizures [5]
Tinnitus
Tremor (<1%)

LEVODOPA

Synonym: L-dopa
Trade name: Sinemet (Bristol-Myers Squibb)
Other common trade names: *Brocadopa; Dopaflex; Dopar; Eldopal; Levodopa-Woelm*
Indications: Parkinsonism
Category: Antidyskinetic; Antiparkinsonian
Half-life: 1–3 hours
Clinically important, potentially hazardous interactions with: kava, MAO inhibitors, phenelzine, pyridoxine, selegiline, tranylcypromine

Sinemet is carbidopa and levodopa

Reactions

Skin
  Diaphoresis [1]
  Exanthems [2]
  Hypomelanosis guttata [1]
  Leukoplakia
  Lupus erythematosus [2]
  Melanoma [26]
  Neuroleptic malignant syndrome [1]
  Pemphigus [1]
  Purpura [1]
  Rash (sic) [2]
  Urticaria
  Vitiligo [1]

Hair
  Hair – alopecia [1]
  Hair – repigmentation [2]

Nails
  Nails – growth [2]

Cardiovascular
  Coronary artery disorders [1]
  Flushing
  Hot flashes

Other
  Ageusia
  Black cartilage [1]
  Bruxism
  Chromhidrosis (1–10%)
  Dysgeusia
  Dyskinesia [9]
  Glossopyrosis
  Headache
  Paresthesias
  Phlebitis
  Priapism
  Sialorrhea
  Xerostomia (1–10%)

LICORICE

Scientific names: *Glycyrrhiza glabra; Glycyrrhiza uralensis*
Family: Fabaceae; Leguminosae
Trade and other common names: Alcazuz; Gan Cao; Gan Zao; Orozuz; Reglisse; Subholz; Sweet Root
Category: Anti-inflammatory
Purported indications and other uses: Upper respiratory tract infection, gastric and duodenal ulcers, bronchitis, colic, dry cough, arthritis, lupus, sore throat, malaria, sores, abscesses, contact dermatitis. Flavoring in foods, beverages and tobacco
Half-life: N/A
Clinically important, potentially hazardous interactions with: cascara, digoxin, hydrocortisone, oral contraceptives, prednisolone

Reactions

Skin
  Dermatitis [1]
  Edema [2]

Cardiovascular
  Hypertension [1]

Other
  Myalgia
  Rhabdomyolysis [16]

LIDOCAINE

Synonym: lignocaine
Trade names: Anamantle HC (Doak); Anestacon; ELA-Max (Ferndale); EMLA (AstraZeneca); Lidoderm (Endo); Xylocaine (AstraZeneca)
Other common trade names: Dentipatch; DermaFlex; Dilocaine; Lidodan; Lidoject-2; Octocaine; Xylocard
Indications: Ventricular arrhythmias, topical anesthesia
Category: Anesthetic; Antiarrhythmic
Half-life: terminal: 1.5–2 hours
Clinically important, potentially hazardous interactions with: amprenavir, antiarrhythmics, cimetidine, fosamprenavir

Reactions

Skin
  Allergic reactions (sic) [1]
  Angioedema [3]
  Bullous eruption
  Dermatitis [25]
  Eczema [3]
  Edema (<1%) [1]

  Erythema [1]
  Erythema multiforme [1]
  Exanthems [2]
  Exfoliative dermatitis [2]
  Fixed eruption [2]
  Lupus erythematosus [1]
  Pigmentation [1]

Pruritus (<1%) [2]
Purpura
Rash (sic) (<1%)
Shivering (1–10%)
Stevens–Johnson syndrome [1]
Urticaria [3]

Other
Acute intermittent porphyria
Anaphylactoid reactions [5]
Application-site edema [1]
Application-site erythema [2]
Application-site pallor [1]

Death [2]
Embolia cutis medicamentosa (Nicolau
  syndrome) [1]
Headache
Hypersensitivity [6]
Injection-site pain
Injection-site phlebitis
Paresthesias (<1%) [1]
Seizures [4]
Stomatitis [1]
Tinnitus
Tremor

LINSEED

Scientific name: *Linum usitatissimum*
Family: Linaceae
Trade and other common names: alpha-linolenic acid; Flaxseed; flaxseed oil; L-310; Igroco;
Lini Semen; linseed oil; lint bells; Salinum; winterlien
Category: Anodyne; Anti-inflammatory; Antiseptic; Antitussive; Demulcent; Emollient;
Expectorant; Laxative; Phytoestrogen
Purported indications and other uses: Dry mouth, menopause, osteoporosis, heart disease,
catarrh, bronchitis, furunculosis, pleuritic pains, constipation, high cholesterol, benign prostatic
hyperplasia, bladder inflammation, gastritis, enteritis, irritable bowel syndrome. **Topical:** poultice
for skin inflammation. **Ophthalmologic:** oil used for removal of foreign bodies from the eye.
Half-life: N/A

Reactions

Skin
Allergic reactions (sic)
Erythema
Irritation

Eyes
Eyelid edema

Other
Anaphylactoid reactions [2]
Fever

Note: Linum is cultivated for both its stem fibers (the source of linen and some paper) and its
seeds (oil used in cooking and in margarine). The oil is used in paints and varnishes and the seed
residues are used in cattle cake

LORAZEPAM

Trade name: Ativan (Wyeth) (Baxter)
Other common trade names: *Apo-Lorazepam; Durazolam; Laubeel; Merlit; Nu-Loraz; Punktyl; Tavor; Temesta; Titus*
Indications: Anxiety, depression
Category: Anticonvulsant; Antiemetic; Benzodiazepine anxiolytic
Half-life: 10–20 hours
Clinically important, potentially hazardous interactions with: alcohol, amprenavir, barbiturates, chlorpheniramine, clarithromycin, CNS depressants, efavirenz, erythromycin, esomeprazole, imatinib, MAO inhibitors, narcotics, nelfinavir, phenothiazines, valproate

Reactions

Skin
  Dermatitis (1–10%)
  Diaphoresis (>10%)
  Erythema multiforme [1]
  Exanthems
  Fixed eruption [1]
  Pruritus
  Purpura
  Rash (sic) (>10%)
  Stevens–Johnson syndrome [1]
  Urticaria

Hair
  Hair – alopecia
  Hair – hirsutism

Cardiovascular
  Bradycardia [1]
  Hypotension [1]

Other
  Gingival lichenoid reaction [1]
  Headache
  Injection-site pain (>10%) [1]
  Injection-site phlebitis (>10%) [1]
  Paresthesias
  Pseudolymphoma [2]
  Rhabdomyolysis [1]
  Sialopenia (>10%)
  Sialorrhea (<1%) [1]
  Tremor (1–10%)
  Xerostomia (>10%)

MAZINDOL

Other common trade names: *Diestet; Liofindol; Solucaps; Teronac*
Indications: Obesity
Category: Anorexiant
Half-life: 10 hours
Clinically important, potentially hazardous interactions with: fluoxetine, fluvoxamine, MAO inhibitors, paroxetine, phenelzine, sertraline, tranylcypromine

Reactions

Skin
  Diaphoresis
  Edema

Exanthems
Rash (sic)
Urticaria

Other
  Dysgeusia

Paresthesias
Xerostomia

MEADOWSWEET

Scientific names: *Filipendula ulmaria; Spiraea ulmaria*
Family: Rosaceae
Trade and other common names: Bridewort; Dolloff; Dropwort; Meadow Queen; Meadow-Wart
Category: Anti-inflammatory; Diuretic
Purported indications and other uses: Colds, fevers, cough, bronchitis, dyspepsia, heartburn, peptic ulcer, gout, rheumatic disorders
Half-life: N/A
Clinically important, potentially hazardous interactions with: salicylates

---

Reactions

Skin
  Rash (sic)

Other
  Hypersensitivity

MECLOFENAMATE

Trade name: Meclofenamate
Other common trade names: *Kyraxan; Melvon; Movens*
Indications: Arthritis
Category: Nonsteroidal anti-inflammatory (NSAID)
Half-life: 2 hours
Clinically important, potentially hazardous interactions with: methotrexate

---

Reactions

Skin
  Angioedema (<1%) [1]
  Bullous eruption
  Edema (>1%)
  Erythema multiforme (<1%) [3]
  Erythema nodosum (<1%)
  Erythroderma [1]
  Exanthems (1–9%) [4]
  Exfoliative dermatitis (<1%) [2]
  Fixed eruption (<1%) [3]
  Lupus erythematosus
  Peripheral edema
  Photosensitivity [2]

  Pruritus (1–10%) [3]
  Psoriasis (exacerbation) [1]
  Purpura (>1%) [4]
  Rash (sic) (3–9%) [1]
  Stevens–Johnson syndrome (<1%)
  Toxic epidermal necrolysis (<1%)
  Urticaria (>1%) [2]
  Vasculitis [3]
  Vesiculobullous eruption [2]

Hair
  Hair – alopecia (<1%)

Cardiovascular
  Hot flashes (<1%)

Other
  Aphthous stomatitis [1]
  Dysgeusia (<1%)
  Headache
  Hypersensitivity [1]

Oral ulceration
Paresthesias (<1%)
Porphyria
Serum sickness
Stomatitis (1–3%)
Tinnitus
Xerostomia

MEFENAMIC ACID

Trade name: Ponstel (First Horizon)
Other common trade names: *Dysman; Lysalgo; Mefac; Mefic; Parkemed; Ponstan; Ponstyl*
Indications: Pain, dysmenorrhea
Category: Nonsteroidal anti-inflammatory (NSAID)
Half-life: 3.5 hours
Clinically important, potentially hazardous interactions with: methotrexate

Reactions

Skin
  Angioedema (<1%)
  Bullous pemphigoid [1]
  Diaphoresis
  Edema
  Erythema multiforme (<1%) [2]
  Exanthems [1]
  Exfoliative dermatitis [1]
  Facial edema
  Fixed eruption [6]
  Photosensitivity [1]
  Pruritus (1–10%)
  Purpura
  Rash (sic) (>10%)
  Stevens–Johnson syndrome (<1%) [1]

Toxic epidermal necrolysis (<1%) [2]
Urticaria (<1%) [1]
Vasculitis [1]

Cardiovascular
  Hot flashes (<1%)

Other
  Anaphylactoid reactions [1]
  Glossitis
  Headache
  Oral ulceration
  Pseudoporphyria [1]
  Sialorrhea
  Xerostomia

MELATONIN

Scientific name: *N-acetyl-5-methoxytryptamine*
Family: None
Trade and other common names: MEL; MLT
Category: Chemoprotectant; Circadian rhythm regulator
Purported indications and other uses: Jet lag, sleep disorders, Alzheimer's disease, free radical scavenger, chemotherapy adjunct, tinnitus, depression, migraine, cluster headache, hypertension, hyperpigmentation, osteoporosis, antioxidant. Skin protectant against sunburn
Half-life: N/A
Clinically important, potentially hazardous interactions with: acetaminophen, NSAIDs, warfarin, zoloft

Reactions

Skin
  Fixed eruption [2]
  Photosensitivity [1]

Other
  Crohn's disease [1]
  Seizures [1]

MELOXICAM

Trade name: Mobic (Boehringer Ingelheim)
Indications: Osteoarthritis
Category: Nonsteroidal anti-inflammatory (NSAID)
Half-life: 15–20 hours

Reactions

Skin
  Adverse effects (sic) (18%) [1]
  Allergic reactions (sic) (<2%)
  Angioedema (<2%) [1]
  Bullous eruption (<2%)
  Edema (2–5%)
  Erythema multiforme (<2%) [1]
  Exanthems (<2%) [3]
  Facial edema [1]
  Peripheral edema [2]
  Photosensitivity (<2%)
  Pruritus (<2%) [2]
  Purpura (<2%)
  Rash (sic) (1–3%) [1]
  Stevens–Johnson syndrome (<2%)

  Toxic epidermal necrolysis (<2%) [1]
  Urticaria (<2%) [1]
  Vasculitis (<2%)

Cardiovascular
  Hot flashes (<2%)

Other
  Anaphylactoid reactions (<2%)
  Dysgeusia (<2%)
  Headache
  Hypersensitivity [1]
  Paresthesias (<2%)
  Tremor (<2%)
  Ulcerative stomatitis (<2%)
  Xerostomia (<2%)

MEPERIDINE

Trade name: Demerol (Sanofi-Aventis)
Other common trade names: *Dolantin; Dolestine; Dolosal; Opistan; Pethidine; Petidin*
Indications: Pain
Category: Narcotic agonist analgesic
Half-life: 3–4 hours
Clinically important, potentially hazardous interactions with: acyclovir, alcohol, amphetamines, barbiturates, CNS depressants, fluoxetine, furazolidone, general anesthetics, isocarboxazid, linezolid, lithium, MAO inhibitors, moclobemide, phenelzine, phenobarbital, phenothiazines, phenytoin, ritonavir, selegiline, sibutramine, SSRIs, tranquilizers, tranylcypromine, tricyclic antidepressants, valacyclovir

Reactions

Skin
  Angioedema [1]
  Diaphoresis
  Herpes [1]
  Necrotizing vasculitis [1]
  Pruritus [3]
  Rash (sic) (<1%)
  Toxic epidermal necrolysis [1]
  Urticaria (<1%) [1]

Cardiovascular
  Flushing

Other
  Cold microabscesses [1]

Dizziness [1]
Embolia cutis medicamentosa (Nicolau syndrome) [1]
Injection-site erythema [2]
Injection-site pain (1–10%)
Injection-site scarring [1]
Injection-site ulceration [1]
Myalgia [1]
Serotonin syndrome [1]
Tremor
Xerostomia (1–10%)

MEPHENYTOIN

Trade name: Mesantoin (Novartis)
Other common trade names: *Epilan-Gerot; Epilanex*
Indications: Partial seizures
Category: Hydantoin anticonvulsant
Half-life: 7 hours (for the active metabolite: 95–144 hours)
Clinically important, potentially hazardous interactions with: chloramphenicol, cyclosporine, disulfiram, dopamine, imatinib, itraconazole

Reactions

Skin
  Acne [1]
  Angioedema [1]

Bullous eruption [1]
Dermatomyositis [1]
Edema

Erythema multiforme [3]
Exanthems (8–10%) [5]
Exfoliative dermatitis [1]
Lupus erythematosus [11]
Pigmentation [4]
Pruritus [1]
Purpura [1]
Scleroderma [1]
Side effects (sic) [1]
Stevens–Johnson syndrome [1]

Toxic epidermal necrolysis [4]
Urticaria [3]

Hair
Hair – alopecia

Other
Gingival hypertrophy
Oral mucosal eruption [1]
Polyarteritis nodosa [1]
Stomatitis [1]

MEPHOBARBITAL

Trade name: Mebaral
Other common trade name: *Prominal*
Indications: Epilepsy, anxiety
Category: Anticonvulsant; Barbiturate ; Sedative
Half-life: 34 hours
Clinically important, potentially hazardous interactions with: alcohol, anticoagulants,
antihistamines, brompheniramine, buclizine, chlorpheniramine, dicumarol, ethanolamine, imatinib,
warfarin

Reactions

Skin
Angioedema (<1%)
Exanthems
Exfoliative dermatitis (<1%)
Purpura
Rash (sic) (<1%)
Stevens–Johnson syndrome (<1%)

Urticaria

Other
Rhabdomyolysis [1]
Serum sickness
Thrombophlebitis (<1%)

METAXALONE

Trade name: Skelaxin (Elan)
Indications: Muscle spasm
Category: Skeletal muscle relaxant
Half-life: 2–3 hours

Reactions

Skin
Dermatitis (<1%)
Fixed eruption [1]
Pruritus
Rash (sic)

Urticaria

Other
Anaphylactoid reactions (<1%)
Headache

METHADONE

Trade name: Dolophine (Roxane)
Other common trade names: *Eptadone; L-Polamidon; Mephenon; Metadon; Methadose; Physeptone*
Indications: Pain, narcotic addiction
Category: Antitussive; Narcotic analgesic; Suppressant (narcotic abstinence syndrome)
Half-life: 15–25 hours
Clinically important, potentially hazardous interactions with: diazepam, erythromycin, fluconazole, fluvoxamine, st john's wort

Reactions

Skin
  Angioedema
  Cellulitis [1]
  Diaphoresis (<48%) [3]
  Exanthems
  Facial edema
  Pruritus (<1%)
  Purpura
  Rash (sic) (<1%)
  Urticaria (<1%)

Cardiovascular
  Flushing

  QT prolongation [1]
  Torsades de pointes [5]

Other
  Death [8]
  Headache
  Injection-site burning
  Injection-site induration
  Injection-site pain (1–10%)
  Rhabdomyolysis [1]
  Tremor [1]
  Xerostomia (1–10%)

METHAMPHETAMINE

Trade name: Desoxyn (Ovation)
Indications: Attention deficit disorder, obesity
Category: Central nervous system stimulant; Recreational drug
Half-life: 4–5 hours
Clinically important, potentially hazardous interactions with: fluoxetine, fluvoxamine, MAO inhibitors, paroxetine, phenelzine, sertraline, tranylcypromine

Reactions

Skin
  Acaraphobia [1]
  Diaphoresis (1–10%)
  Lichenoid eruption [1]
  Nodular eruption [1]
  Pigmentation [1]
  Rash (sic) (<1%)

  Toxic epidermal necrolysis [1]
  Urticaria (<1%)

Cardiovascular
  Angina [1]

Other
  Anxiety [1]
  Death [2]

Delusions of parasitosis [1]
Depression [1]
Dysgeusia
Gynecomastia [1]
Headache

Injection-site lipoatrophy [1]
Polyarteritis nodosa [2]
Rhabdomyolysis (43%) [5]
Tremor
Xerostomia (1–10%)

METHANTHELINE

Other common trade name: *Vagantin*
Indications: Duodenal ulcer
Category: Gastrointestinal anticholinergic
Half-life: N/A
Clinically important, potentially hazardous interactions with: anticholinergics, arbutamine

Reactions

Skin
Exanthems
Exfoliative dermatitis
Hypohidrosis
Urticaria
Xerosis

Cardiovascular
Flushing

Other
Ageusia
Anaphylactoid reactions
Dysgeusia
Sialopenia
Xerostomia

METHENAMINE

Trade names: Hiprex (Sanofi-Aventis); Mandelamine; Prosed; Urised; Uroqid
Other common trade names: *Dehydral; Haiprex; Hip-Rex; Hipeksal; Hippramine; Reflux; Urasal; Urotractan*
Indications: Urinary tract infections
Category: Urinary tract antibacterial
Half-life: 3–6 hours

Reactions

Skin
Dermatitis (systemic)
Edema
Erythema multiforme (<1%)
Exanthems (<1%) [2]
Fixed eruption (<1%) [1]
Photosensitivity [1]

Pruritus (<1%)
Rash (sic) (3.5%)
Urticaria

Other
Headache
Stomatitis

METHOCARBAMOL

Trade name: Robaxin (Baxter) (Elkins-Sinn)
Other common trade names: *Carbametin; Carxin; Delaxin; Lumirelax; Marbaxin; Miowas; Ortoton; Robinax; Robomol; Trolar*
Indications: Muscle spasm, tetanus
Category: Skeletal muscle relaxant
Half-life: 1–2 hours

Reactions

Skin
  Allergic reactions (sic) (1–10%)
  Exanthems
  Pruritus
  Rash (sic)
  Urticaria

Cardiovascular
  Flushing (1–10%)

Other
  Anaphylactoid reactions
  Dysgeusia
  Headache
  Injection-site pain (<1%)
  Thrombophlebitis (<1%)

METHOTREXATE

Synonyms: amethopterin; MTX
Trade name: Rheumatrex (Stada)
Other common trade names: *Farmitrexat; Lantarel; Ledertrexate; Maxtrex; Metex; Texate*
Indications: Carcinomas, leukemias, lymphomas, psoriasis, rheumatoid arthritis
Category: Anti-inflammatory; Antiarthritic; Antineoplastic
Half-life: 3–10 hours
Clinically important, potentially hazardous interactions with: acitretin, aldesleukin, aminoglycosides, amiodarone, amoxicillin, ampicillin, aspirin, bacampicillin, bismuth, carbenicillin, chloroquine, cisplatin, cloxacillin, co-trimoxazole, dapsone, demeclocycline, diclofenac, dicloxacillin, etodolac, etretinate, fenoprofen, flurbiprofen, folic acid antagonists, haloperidol, ibuprofen, indomethacin, influenza vaccines, ketoprofen, ketorolac, lithium, magnesium trisalicylate, meclofenamate, mefenamic acid, methicillin, mezlocillin, minocycline, nabumetone, nafcillin, naproxen, NSAIDs, omeprazole, oxacillin, oxaprozin, oxytetracycline, paromomycin, penicillins, piperacillin, piroxicam, polypeptide antibiotics, probenecid, procarbazine, rofecoxib, salicylates, salsalate, sulfadiazine, sulfamethoxazole, sulfapyridine, sulfasalazine, sulfisoxazole, sulindac, tetracycline, ticarcillin, tolmetin, trimethoprim, vaccines

Reactions

Skin
  Acne
  Acral erythema [4]
  Allergic reactions (sic) [1]

  Bullous eruption [2]
  Burning (palms and soles) [1]
  Candidiasis [1]
  Capillaritis [2]

Carcinoma [1]
Dermatitis [1]
Eccrine squamous syringometaplasia [1]
Edema [1]
Erosion of psoriatic plaques [8]
Erosions [1]
Erythema (>10%)
Erythema multiforme [3]
Erythroderma [2]
Exanthems (15%) [3]
Folliculitis [1]
Furunculosis [1]
Herpes simplex [1]
Inflammation (reactivation) [1]
Melanoma [1]
Necrosis [4]
Nodular eruption [11]
Photo-recall [4]
Photosensitivity (5%) [7]
Pigmentation (1–10%)
Pruritus (1–5%) [1]
Purpura
Radiodermatitis (reactivation)
Rash (sic) (1–3%) [2]
Scabies (reactivation) [1]
Side effects (sic) [2]
Squamous cell carcinoma [2]
Stevens–Johnson syndrome [3]
Sunburn (reactivation) [5]
Telangiectasia
Toxic epidermal necrolysis (<1%) [4]
Ulceration of psoriatic plaques [1]
Ulcerations [7]
Urticaria [4]

Vasculitis (>10%) [8]

Hair
Hair – alopecia (1–6%) [12]
Hair – pigmented bands [1]

Nails
Nails – discoloration
Nails – onycholysis [1]
Nails – paronychia [1]
Nails – pigmentation [1]

Hematopoietic
Ecchymoses [1]

Other
Anaphylactoid reactions (1–10%) [6]
Death
Dysgeusia [1]
Gingivitis (>10%)
Glossitis (>10%)
Gynecomastia [3]
Headache
Hodgkin's disease (nodular sclerosing) [1]
Hypersensitivity [1]
Malignant lymphoma [4]
Mucositis [1]
Myalgia
Oral mucositis [5]
Oral ulceration [5]
Peyronie's disease [1]
Porphyria cutanea tarda [1]
Pseudolymphoma [10]
Stomatitis (3–10%) [7]
Tendinitis [1]
Tinnitus

METHOXYFLURANE

Trade name: Penthrane (Abbott) (Ger)
Indications: Anesthesia
Category: Anesthesia adjunct
Half-life: N/A
Clinically important, potentially hazardous interactions with: cisatracurium, demeclocycline, doxacurium, doxycycline, gentamicin, kanamycin, minocycline, neomycin, oxytetracycline, pancuronium, rapacuronium, streptomycin, tetracycline

METHSUXIMIDE

Trade name: Celontin (Pfizer)
Other common trade name: *Petinutin*
Indications: Absence (petit-mal) seizures
Category: Succinimide anticonvulsant
Half-life: 2–4 hours

Reactions

Skin
  Acanthosis nigricans [1]
  Erythema multiforme
  Exanthems [1]
  Exfoliative dermatitis (<1%)
  Lupus erythematosus (>10%)
  Pruritus
  Purpura
  Rash (sic)
  Stevens–Johnson syndrome (>10%)
  Urticaria (<1%)

Hair
  Hair – alopecia
  Hair – hirsutism

Eyes
  Periorbital edema

Other
  Gingival hypertrophy
  Headache
  Oral ulceration

METHYLPHENIDATE

Trade names: Concerta; Metadate CD (Celltech); Methylin (Mallinckrodt); Ritalin (Novartis)
Other common trade names: *Centedrin; Rilatine; Rubifen*
Indications: Attention deficit disorder, narcolepsy
Category: Central nervous system stimulant
Half-life: 2–4 hours
Clinically important, potentially hazardous interactions with: cyclosporine, pimozide

Reactions

Skin
  Angioedema [2]
  Diaphoresis
  Erythema multiforme
  Exanthems [1]
  Exfoliative dermatitis [2]
  Fixed eruption [1]
  Photosensitivity [1]
  Pruritus
  Purpura [1]
  Rash (sic) (<1%)
  Urticaria [1]

  Vasculitis [1]

Hair
  Hair – alopecia

Eyes
  Eyelid edema [1]

Cardiovascular
  QT prolongation [1]

Other
  Anxiety [1]
  Bruxism [1]

Delusions of parasitosis [1]
Depression [1]
Dyskinesia [1]
Headache
Hypersensitivity (1–10%) [1]

Injection-site abscess [1]
Sialorrhea [1]
Tourette's syndrome
Xerostomia [2]

METHYSERGIDE

Trade name: Sansert (Novartis)
Other common trade names: *Deseril; Desernil; Deserril; Deseryl*
Indications: Vascular (migraine) headaches
Category: Ergot alkaloid; Vascular headache prophylactic
Half-life: 10 hours
Clinically important, potentially hazardous interactions with: almotriptan, amprenavir, clarithromycin, delavirdine, efavirenz, erythromycin, indinavir, naratriptan, nelfinavir, ritonavir, rizatriptan, saquinavir, sibutramine, sumatriptan, troleandomycin, zolmitriptan

---

Reactions

Skin
  Adverse effects (sic) [1]
  Collagen disease [1]
  Exanthems
  Hypermelanosis [1]
  Lupus erythematosus [2]
  Orange-peel skin [1]
  Peripheral edema (1–10%)
  Pruritus
  Rash (sic) (1–10%)
  Raynaud's phenomenon
  Scleroderma [3]
  Telangiectasia

Urticaria

Hair
  Hair – alopecia [4]

Cardiovascular
  Flushing [1]
  Myocarditis [1]

Other
  Headache
  Hyperesthesia (<1%)
  Myalgia
  Paresthesias

MILK THISTLE*

Scientific names: *Carduus marainum; Silibum marianum*
Family: Asteraceae; Compositae
Trade and other common names: Holy Thistle; Lady's Thistle; Marian Thistle; Mary Thistle; Silymarin
Category: Anti-inflammatory; Anticancer; Hepatoprotective
Purported indications and other uses: Dyspepsia, liver protectant, hepatitis, loss of appetite, spleen diseases, supportive treatment for mushroom poisoning
Half-life: N/A

Reactions

Skin

Adverse effects (sic) [2]
Allergic reactions (sic)

Diaphoresis
Rash (sic) [1]
Urticaria [1]

*Note: Seed as opposed to the 'aboveground parts'

MISTLETOE

Scientific names: *Phoradendron flavescens; Phoradendron leucarpum; Phoradendron macrophyllum; Phoradendron rubrum; Phoradendron serotinum; Phoradendron tomentosum; Viscum album*
Family: Loranthacae; Viscaceae
Trade and other common names: ABNOBA viscum; All-heal; Devil's fuge; Eurixor; Folia Visci; Helixor; Herbe de la Croix; Iscador (Weleda); Isorel (Novipharm); Lektinol; Lignum Crucis; Stipites Visci; VaQuFrF (Labor Hiscia); Vysorel
Category: Adjuvant; Immune modulator
Purported indications and other uses: Injected: adjuvant tumor therapy. **Oral:** abortifacient, arteriosclerosis, arthritis, asthma, colds, depression, headache, HIV infection, hypertension, hypotension, hysteria, labor pain, lumbago, metrorrhagia, muscle spasms, otitis, whooping cough, hemorrhoids, internal bleeding, gout, sleep disorders, amenorrhea, liver and gallbladder conditions
Half-life: N/A
Clinically important, potentially hazardous interactions with: bepridil, corticosteroids, digoxin, diltiazem, immunosuppressants, MAO inhibitors, verapamil

Note: Purified extracts injected intramuscularly, subcutaneously or by intravenous infusion. Unless otherwise indicated, side effects listed are from injected preparations. The FDA considers *Viscum album* unsafe

Reactions

Skin

Adverse effects (sic) [2]
Allergic reactions (sic) [3]
Chills [2]
Dermatitis [1]
Edema of lip [1]
Erythema [3]
Flu-like syndrome [2]
Nodular eruption [1]

Pruritus [1]

Other

Anaphylactoid reactions (28%) [2]
Death (low incidence – accidental ingestion) [4]
Gingivitis [2]
Injection-site edema [1]
Injection-site inflammation [6]

*Note: The well-known mistletoe is an evergreen parasitic plant, growing on the branches of some tree species

**Note: Shakespeare calls it 'the baleful mistletoe,' an illusion to the Scandinavian legend that Balder, the god of Peace, was slain with an arrow made of mistletoe

MODAFINIL

Trade name: Provigil (Cephalon)
Other common trade name: Alertec
Indications: Narcolepsy
Category: Analeptic; Central nervous system stimulant
Half-life: ~15 hours
Clinically important, potentially hazardous interactions with: oral contraceptives

Reactions

Skin
Allergic reactions (sic) (>1%)
Chills (2%)
Diaphoresis (>1%)
Edema (>1%)
Erythema
Herpes simplex (1%)
Pruritus (>1%)
Psoriasis (>1%)
Rash (sic) (>1%)
Xerosis (1%)

Hematopoietic
Ecchymoses (>1%)

Cardiovascular
Hot flashes

Other
Anxiety (16%) [1]
Dizziness [1]
Dysgeusia (>1%)
Gingivitis (1%)
Headache (28%) [1]
Myalgia (>1%)
Oral ulceration (1%)
Paresthesias (3%) [1]
Sialorrhea
Tooth disorder (sic) (>1%)
Tremor (1%)
Xerostomia (5%)

MORPHINE

Trade names: Astramorph; Avinza (Ligand); Duramorph (Baxter) (Elkins-Sinn); Infumorph (Baxter); Kadian (aaiPharma); MS Contin (Purdue); MS/S; MSIR Oral (Purdue); OMS Oral; Oramorph SR; RMS; Roxanol (aaiPharma)
Other common trade names: Anamorph; Astramorph; Contalgin; Epimorph; Morphine-HP; MOS; Moscontin; MS-IR; MST Continus; Sevredol; Statex
Indications: Severe pain, acute myocardial infarction
Category: Narcotic analgesic
Half-life: 2–4 hours
Clinically important, potentially hazardous interactions with: buprenorphine, cimetidine, furazolidone, MAO inhibitors, pentazocine

Reactions

Skin
Diaphoresis [1]

Edema
Exanthems [1]

Pallor

Peripheral edema

Pruritus (5–65%) [17]

Pustular psoriasis [1]

Rash (sic)

Cardiovascular

Bradycardia [1]

Flushing

Hypotension [1]

Other

Death [1]

Gynecomastia

Hyperalgesia [1]

Hyperesthesia

Injection-site pain (>10%)

Rhabdomyolysis [2]

Trembling (1–10%)

Xerostomia (>10%) [2]

MYRRH

Scientific names: *Commiphora abyssinica; Commiphora erythraea; Commiphora habessinica; Commiphora kataf; Commiphora madagascariensis; Commiphora molmol; Commiphora myrrh*

Family: Burseraceae

Trade and other common names: Bal; Balsamodendron; Bdellium; Bol; Bola; Didin; Didthin; Heerabol; Mirazid; Mirra; Morr

Category: Anesthetic; Anti-inflammatory; Antibacterial; Antifungal; Astringent; Carminative; Emmenagogue; Expectorant; Vermifuge

Purported indications and other uses: Fascioliasis, schistosomiasis, ulcers, eczema, catarrh, amenorrhoea, gum disease, aphthous stomatitis

Half-life: N/A

Clinically important, potentially hazardous interactions with: methimazole, propylthiouracil

Reactions

Skin

Dermatitis [5]

Pruritus (0.5%) [1]

Side effects (sic) [1]

Other

Abdominal pain (2%) [1]

Fatigue (2.5%) [1]

Headache (0.5%) [1]

Rhabdomyolysis [1]

*Note: no interactions have been reported. The drugs listed may interact

NABUMETONE

Trade name: Relafen (GSK)
Other common trade names: *Arthaxan; Consolan; Nabuser; Prodac; Relif; Relifex; Unimetone*
Indications: Arthritis
Category: Nonsteroidal anti-inflammatory (NSAID)
Half-life: 22.5–30 hours
Clinically important, potentially hazardous interactions with: methotrexate

Reactions

Skin
  Acne (<1%)
  Adverse effects (sic) [1]
  Angioedema (<1%) [1]
  Bullous eruption (<1%)
  Diaphoresis (1–3%)
  Edema (3–9%) [1]
  Erythema [1]
  Erythema multiforme (<1%)
  Exanthems (1.2%) [2]
  Photosensitivity (<1%) [5]
  Phototoxicity [1]
  Pruritus (3–9%) [2]
  Rash (sic) (3–9%) [4]
  Side effects (sic) [1]
  Stevens–Johnson syndrome (<1%) [1]
  Toxic epidermal necrolysis (<1%)
  Urticaria (<1%)
  Vasculitis (necrotizing) [1]
  Xerosis [1]

Hair
  Hair – alopecia (<1%) [1]

Cardiovascular
  Hot flashes (<1%)

Other
  Anaphylactoid reactions (<1%)
  Gingivitis (<1%)
  Glossitis (<1%)
  Headache
  Myalgia
  Oral ulceration [1]
  Paresthesias (<1%)
  Parkinsonism
  Porphyria cutanea tarda (<1%)
  Pseudolymphoma [1]
  Pseudoporphyria [6]
  Sialorrhea
  Stomatitis (1–3%)
  Tinnitus
  Xerostomia (1–3%)

NADOLOL

Trade names: Corgard; Corzide (Monarch)
Other common trade names: *Apo-Nadolol; Farmagard; Nadic; Solgol; Syn-Nadolol*
Indications: Hypertension, angina pectoris
Category: Antianginal; Antihypertensive; Beta-adrenoceptor blocker
Half-life: 10–24 hours
Clinically important, potentially hazardous interactions with: clonidine, epinephrine, verapamil

Corzide is nadolol and bendroflumethiazide*

Note: Cutaneous side effects of beta-receptor blockaders are clinically polymorphous. They apparently appear after several months of continuous therapy. Atypical psoriasiform, lichen planus-like, and eczematous chronic rashes are mainly observed. (1983): Hödl St, *Z Hautkr* (German) 58, 17

Reactions

Skin
Bullous pemphigoid [1]
Diaphoresis (< 1%) [1]
Eczema
Edema (1–5%)
Erythema multiforme
Exanthems (< 1%) [1]
Exfoliative dermatitis
Facial edema (< 1%)
Hyperkeratosis (palms and soles)
Infiltrative dermatitis of the scalp [1]
Lichenoid eruption [1]
Lupus erythematosus
Pityriasis rubra pilaris [1]
Pruritus (1–5%)
Psoriasis [4]
Pustules [1]
Rash (sic) (1–5%)
Raynaud's phenomenon (2%) [2]
Toxic epidermal necrolysis
Urticaria

Xerosis

Hair
Hair – alopecia [1]

Nails
Nails – dystrophy
Nails – onycholysis
Nails – pigmentation

Eyes
Oculo-mucocutaneous syndrome [1]

Other
Dysgeusia
Gingivitis [1]
Headache
Numbness (fingers and toes) (>5%)
Oral lichenoid eruption
Oral mucosal eruption (< 1%) [1]
Paresthesias (>5%)
Peyronie's disease [1]
Tinnitus
Xerostomia (< 1%) [1]

*Note: Bendroflumethiazide is a sulfonamide and can be absorbed systemically. Sulfonamides can produce severe, possibly fatal, reactions such as toxic epidermal necrolysis and Stevens–Johnson syndrome

NALBUPHINE

Trade name: Nubain (Endo)
Other common trade names: *Bufigen; Nalcryn SP; Nubain SP*
Indications: Moderate to severe pain
Category: Narcotic agonist-antagonistic analgesic
Half-life: 5 hours
Clinically important, potentially hazardous interactions with: CNS depressants, diazepam, pentobarbital, promethazine

Note: Nalbuphine contains sulfites

Reactions

Skin
  Burning (<1%) [1]
  Clammy skin (9%)
  Diaphoresis (9%)
  Pruritus (<1%)
  Urticaria (<1%)

Eyes
  Blurred vision

Cardiovascular
  Flushing (<1%)

Other
  Depression (<1%)
  Dizziness (5%) [1]
  Dysgeusia (<1%)
  Headache
  Injection-site pain [2]
  Numbness
  Paresthesias
  Tingling
  Xerostomia (4%)

NAPROXEN

Trade names: Aleve; Naprosyn (Roche)
Other common trade names: *Aleve; Anaprox; Apranax; Dymenalgit; Flanax; Laraflex; Naprelan; Naprogesic; Napron X; Naprosyne; Naxen; Novo-Naprox; Nu-Naprox; Supradol; Synflex; Velsay*
Indications: Pain, arthritis
Category: Nonsteroidal anti-inflammatory (NSAID)
Half-life: 13 hours
Clinically important, potentially hazardous interactions with: boswellia, methotrexate

Reactions

Skin
  Angioedema (<1%) [2]
  Baboon syndrome [1]
  Bullous eruption [5]
  Diaphoresis (<3%) [3]
  Edema (1–9%) [1]
  Erythema multiforme (<1%) [2]
  Erythema nodosum [1]

  Exanthems (1–14%) [10]
  Exfoliative dermatitis
  Facial scarring [1]
  Fixed eruption [15]
  Lichen planus [3]
  Lichenoid eruption [3]
  Linear IgA dermatosis [1]
  Lupus erythematosus [1]

Peripheral edema [1]
Photosensitivity (bullous) [1]
Photosensitivity (<1%) [14]
Phototoxicity [1]
Pityriasis rosea [1]
Pruritus (3–17%) [6]
Pseudoreactions [1]
Purpura (<3%) [4]
Pustules [2]
Pyogenic granuloma [1]
Rash (sic) (3–9%) [2]
Side effects (sic) (5–9%) [3]
Stevens–Johnson syndrome (<1%)
Toxic epidermal necrolysis (<1%) [1]
Urticaria (1–5%) [6]
Vasculitis [9]
Vesiculobullous eruption [1]

Hair
Hair – alopecia (<1%) [3]

Hematopoietic
Ecchymoses (3–9%)

Cardiovascular
Hot flashes (<1%)

Other
Anaphylactoid reactions (<1%)
Aphthous stomatitis [1]
Headache
Hypersensitivity [1]
Myalgia (<1%)
Oral ulceration [1]
Porphyria cutanea tarda [1]
Pseudolymphoma [1]
Pseudoporphyria [27]
Salivary gland enlargement [1]
Stomatitis (<3%)
Tinnitus
Xerostomia

NARATRIPTAN

Trade name: Amerge (GSK)
Indications: Acute migraine attacks
Category: Antimigraine; Serotonin agonist
Half-life: 6 hours
Clinically important, potentially hazardous interactions with: dihydroergotamine,
ergotamine, methysergide, rizatriptan, sibutramine, st john's wort, sumatriptan, zolmitriptan

---

Reactions

Skin
Acne (<1%)
Allergic reactions (sic) (<1%)
Dermatitis (<1%)
Diaphoresis (<1%)
Edema (<1%)
Erythema (<1%)
Exanthems (<1%)
Folliculitis (<1%)
Photosensitivity (<1%)
Purpura (<1%)
Rash (sic) (<1%)
Sensitivity (sic) (<1)%

Urticaria (<1%)
Xerosis (<1%)

Hair
Hair – alopecia (<1%)

Eyes
Ocular pigmentation (<1%)

Other
Dysgeusia (<1%)
Headache
Hyperesthesia (<1%)
Paresthesias (2%)
Sialopenia (<1%)

NICARDIPINE

Trade name: Cardene (Roche)
Other common trade names: *Antagonil; Dagan; Loxen; Nicardal; Nicodel; Ranvil; Ridene; Rydene*
Indications: Angina, hypertension
Category: Antianginal; Antimigraine; Calcium channel blocker
Half-life: 2–4 hours
Clinically important, potentially hazardous interactions with: epirubicin, imatinib, telithromycin

---

Reactions

Skin
 Allergic reactions (sic)
 Edema (1%)
 Exanthems
 Peripheral edema (7.1%) [2]
 Rash (sic) (1.2%) [3]
 Side effects (sic) [1]
 Urticaria [3]

Cardiovascular
 Flushing (5.6%) [2]

Other
 Erythromelalgia [2]
 Gingival hypertrophy (<1%)
 Headache
 Myalgia (1%) [1]
 Paresthesias (1%)
 Parotitis
 Tinnitus
 Xerostomia (1.4%)

NIFEDIPINE

Trade names: Adalat (Bayer); Procardia (Pfizer)
Other common trade names: *Adalate; Apo-Nifed; Aprical; Calcilat; Coracten; Corogal; Corotrend; Nifecor; Nu-Nifed; Pidilat*
Indications: Angina, hypertension
Category: Antianginal; Antimigraine; Calcium channel blocker
Half-life: 2–5 hours
Clinically important, potentially hazardous interactions with: epirubicin, grapefruit juice, imatinib, rifampin, ritonavir

---

Reactions

Skin
 Acute generalized exanthematous
  pustulosis (AGEP) [2]
 Angioedema (<1%) [2]
 Bullous eruption [2]
 Chills (2%)
 Dermatitis (<2%)
 Diaphoresis (<2%) [2]

 Edema [2]
 Erysipelas [2]
 Erythema [2]
 Erythema multiforme [4]
 Erythema nodosum [2]
 Exanthems (1%) [9]
 Exfoliative dermatitis (<1%) [5]
 Facial edema (1%)

Fixed eruption [3]
Lichenoid eruption [3]
Lupus erythematosus [3]
Pemphigoid nodularis [1]
Pemphigus foliaceus [1]
Peripheral edema [8]
Photosensitivity [6]
Prurigo nodularis [1]
Pruritus (<2%) [3]
Purpura (<2%) [3]
Rash (sic) (<3%) [2]
Shaking (2%)
Side effects (sic) [1]
Stevens–Johnson syndrome [3]
Telangiectasia [3]
Toxic epidermal necrolysis [2]
Ulcerations [1]
Urticaria (<1%) [7]
Vasculitis [3]

Hair
Hair – alopecia (1%) [4]
Hair – pigmentation [1]

Nails
Nails – dystrophy [1]

Eyes
Periorbital edema (1%) [1]

Cardiovascular
Angina [1]
Flushing (3–25%) [5]

Other
Dysgeusia (<1%)
Erythromelalgia (<0.5%) [4]
Gingival hypertrophy (6–10%) [39]
Gynecomastia (<1%) [3]
Headache
Myalgia (<1%)
Paresthesias (<3%) [1]
Parosmia
Parotitis
Tinnitus
Tremor (2–8%)
Xerostomia (<3%)

NITROGLYCERIN

Synonyms: glyceryl trinitrate; nitroglycerol; NTG

Trade names:

Buccal tablets

Lingual aerosol: Nitrolingual (First Horizon)

Oral capsules: Nitrocap; Nitrocine; Nitroglyn; Nitrospan

Oral tablets: Klavikordal; Niong; Nitronet; Nitrong

Parenteral: Nitro-Bid; Nitroject; Nitrol; Nitrostat (Pfizer); Tridil

Sublingual tablets: Nitrostat (Pfizer)

Topical ointment: Nitrol; Nitrong; Nitrostat (Pfizer)

Topical transdermal systems: Deponit; Minitran (3M); Nitrocine; Nitrodisc; Nitrodur; Transderm-Nitro (Various pharmaceutical companies.)

Other common trade names: *Cardinit; Corditrine; Lenitral; Nitrodisc; Nitroglin; Suscard; Sustac*
Indications: Acute angina
Category: Antianginal; Antihypertensive; Vasodilator
Half-life: 1–4 minutes
Clinically important, potentially hazardous interactions with: acetylcysteine, alteplase, sildenafil

Reactions

Skin

Allergic reactions (sic) (<1%)

Angioedema [1]

Cyanosis

Dermatitis (to topical systems) (<1%) [23]

Diaphoresis (<1%)

Eczema [2]

Edema

Erythema (to transdermal delivery system) [2]

Erythema multiforme [1]

Erythroderma [1]

Exanthems

Exfoliative dermatitis (1–10%) [1]

Irritation [1]

Pallor

Peripheral edema (<1%)

Purpura [2]

Rash (sic) (1–10%)

Rosacea (exacerbation) [1]

Urticaria

Cardiovascular

Bradycardia [1]

Flushing (>10%) [1]

Hypotension [1]

Other

Anaphylactoid reactions (from perianal application) [1]

Headache [2]

Oral burn (from sublingual)

Systemic reactions [1]

Xerostomia (<1%)

NORTRIPTYLINE

Trade names: Aventyl (Ranbaxy); Pamelor (Mallinckrodt)
Other common trade names: *Allegron; Apo-Nortriptyline; Noritren; Norpress; Nortrilen; Paxtibi; Vividyl*
Indications: Depression
Category: Tricyclic antidepressant
Half-life: 28–31 hours
Clinically important, potentially hazardous interactions with: amprenavir, arbutamine, clonidine, epinephrine, fluoxetine, formoterol, guanethidine, isocarboxazid, linezolid, MAO inhibitors, phenelzine, quinolones, sparfloxacin, tranylcypromine

Reactions

Skin
  Acne
  Allergic reactions (sic) (<1%)
  Diaphoresis (1–10%)
  Edema
  Erythema
  Exanthems
  Petechiae
  Photosensitivity (<1%) [2]
  Phototoxicity
  Pruritus
  Purpura
  Rash (sic)
  Urticaria
  Vasculitis
  Xerosis

Hair
  Hair – alopecia (<1%)

Cardiovascular
  Flushing
  QT prolongation [1]

Other
  Acute intermittent porphyria [1]
  Black tongue [1]
  Dizziness [1]
  Dysgeusia (>10%)
  Galactorrhea (<1%)
  Gynecomastia (<1%)
  Paresthesias
  Parkinsonism (1–10%)
  Stomatitis
  Tinnitus
  Tongue edema
  Tremor
  Vaginitis
  Xerostomia (>10%) [2]

OMEPRAZOLE

Trade name: Prilosec (AstraZeneca)
Other common trade names: *Antra; Audazol; Gastroloc; Inhibitron; Logastric; Losec; Mopral; Omed; Ozoken; Parizac; Ulsen*
Indications: Duodenal ulcer, Gastroesophageal Reflux Disease (GERD)
Category: Antiulcer; Gastric acid secretion inhibitor; Proton pump inhibitor
Half-life: 0.5–1 hour
Clinically important, potentially hazardous interactions with: eucalyptus, methotrexate

Reactions

Skin
  Angioedema (<1%) [3]
  Baboon syndrome [1]
  Bullous eruption [1]
  Bullous pemphigoid [2]
  Burning [1]
  Dermatitis [1]
  Diaphoresis (<1%) [1]
  Eczema [1]
  Edema (1–10%) [2]
  Erythema [1]
  Erythema multiforme (<1%)
  Erythema nodosum [1]
  Erythroderma [1]
  Exanthems [1]
  Exfoliative dermatitis [2]
  Facial edema [1]
  Fixed eruption [1]
  Furunculosis [1]
  Lichen planus [3]
  Lichen spinulosus [2]
  Lichenoid eruption [1]
  Lupus erythematosus [1]
  Pemphigus (exacerbation) [2]
  Peripheral edema (<1%) [2]
  Pityriasis rosea [1]
  Pruritus (1–10%) [8]
  Psoriasis [1]
  Purpura
  Rash (sic) (1.5%) [5]
  Stevens–Johnson syndrome (<1%)
  Toxic epidermal necrolysis (<1%) [2]
  Urticaria (1–10%) [6]
  Vasculitis [1]
  Xerosis (<1%) [1]

Hair
  Hair – alopecia (<1%) [4]
  Hair – pigmentation

Eyes
  Periorbital edema [1]

Other
  Anaphylactoid reactions [3]
  Cough [1]
  Dysesthesia (<1%)
  Dysgeusia (1–10%) [1]
  Gynecomastia [9]
  Headache
  Myalgia (1–10%)
  Oral candidiasis [3]
  Paresthesias (<1%) [2]
  Tinnitus
  Tremor (<1%)
  Xerostomia (1–10%) [1]

ONDANSETRON

Trade name: Zofran (GSK)
Other common trade names: *Emeset; Oncoden; Zofron*
Indications: Nausea and vomiting
Category: Antiemetic; Serotonin antagonist
Half-life: 4 hours
Clinically important, potentially hazardous interactions with: eucalyptus

Reactions

Skin
 Angioedema
 Chills (5–10%)
 Exanthems
 Fixed eruption [2]
 Pruritus (5%)
 Rash (sic) (<1%)
 Urticaria

Hair
 Hair – alopecia

Cardiovascular
 Flushing [1]
 QT prolongation [1]

Other
 Anaphylactoid reactions [3]
 Dysgeusia [1]
 Headache
 Hypersensitivity (<1%) [1]
 Injection-site burning
 Injection-site erythema
 Injection-site pain
 Injection-site reactions (sic) (4%)
 Paresthesias (2%)
 Porphyria [1]
 Sialopenia (1–5%)
 Xerostomia (1–10%) [2]

ORPHENADRINE

Trade names: Banflex (Forest); Norflex (3M)
Other common trade names: *Biorfen; Biorphen; Disipal; Distalene; Flexojet; Flexon; Myolin; Norgesic; Opheryl; Orfenace; Prolongatum*
Indications: Painful musculoskeletal conditions
Category: Skeletal muscle relaxant
Half-life: 14 hours

Reactions

Skin
 Exanthems
 Fixed eruption [1]
 Pigmentation [1]
 Pruritus
 Rash (sic) (1–10%)
 Urticaria

Cardiovascular
 Flushing (1–10%)

Other
 Anaphylactoid reactions
 Embolia cutis medicamentosa (Nicolau
   syndrome) [1]
 Headache
 Hypersensitivity
 Paresthesias
 Xerostomia

OXAPROZIN

Trade name: Daypro (Pfizer)
Other common trade names: *Deflam; Duraprox*
Indications: Arthritis
Category: Nonsteroidal anti-inflammatory (NSAID)
Half-life: 42–50 hours
Clinically important, potentially hazardous interactions with: methotrexate

Reactions

Skin
  Angioedema (<1%)
  Diaphoresis (<1%)
  Edema (<1%)
  Erythema
  Erythema multiforme (<1%) [1]
  Exanthems [4]
  Exfoliative dermatitis (<1%)
  Fixed eruption [1]
  Linear IgA dermatosis [1]
  Photosensitivity (<1%)
  Phototoxicity [2]
  Pruritus (1–10%) [1]
  Purpura
  Rash (sic) (>10%) [2]
  Stevens–Johnson syndrome (<1%) [1]
  Toxic epidermal necrolysis [3]
  Urticaria (<1%) [1]

  Vasculitis [1]
Hair
  Hair – alopecia
Hematopoietic
  Ecchymoses (<1%)
Other
  Anaphylactoid reactions (<1%)
  Death
  Dysgeusia
  Headache
  Pseudolymphoma [1]
  Pseudoporphyria [3]
  Serum sickness (<1%)
  Stomatitis (<1%)
  Tinnitus

OXAZEPAM

Trade name: Serax (Mayne)
Other common trade names: *Adumbran; Apo-Oxazepam; Azutranquil; Durazepam; Murelax; Novoxapam; Oxpam; Praxiten; Serax; Serepax; Zapex*
Indications: Anxiety, depression
Category: Anticonvulsant; Benzodiazepine sedative-hypnotic
Half-life: 3–6 hours
Clinically important, potentially hazardous interactions with: amprenavir, chlorpheniramine, clarithromycin, efavirenz, esomeprazole, imatinib, nelfinavir

Reactions

Skin
  Dermatitis (1–10%)

  Diaphoresis (>10%)
  Edema

Erythema multiforme [1]
Exanthems
Fixed eruption [1]
Pruritus
Purpura
Rash (sic) (>10%)
Toxic epidermal necrolysis [1]
Urticaria

Other
  Headache
  Paresthesias
  Sialopenia (>10%)
  Sialorrhea (1–10%)
  Tongue furry
  Tremor
  Xerostomia (>10%)

OXCARBAZEPINE

Synonym: GP 47680
Trade name: Trileptal (Novartis)
Indications: Partial epileptic seizures
Category: Anticonvulsant
Half-life: 1–2.5 hours

Reactions

Skin
  Acne
  Allergic reactions (sic) (2%) [2]
  Angioedema
  Dermatitis
  Diaphoresis (3%)
  Eczema
  Edema (2%)
  Erythema multiforme
  Exanthems [2]
  Facial rash (sic)
  Folliculitis
  Genital pruritus
  Infections (2%)
  Lupus erythematosus
  Photosensitivity
  Purpura (2%)
  Rash (sic) (<6%) [1]
  Sensitivity [1]
  Stevens–Johnson syndrome
  Toxic epidermal necrolysis

  Vitiligo
Hair
  Hair – alopecia

Cardiovascular
  Hot flashes (2%)

Other
  Dysgeusia (5%)
  Gingival hypertrophy
  Headache
  Hyperesthesia (3%)
  Hypersensitivity [1]
  Oral ulceration [1]
  Priapism
  Stomatitis
  Toothache (2%)
  Tremor (4–6%)
  Ulcerative stomatitis
  Vaginitis (2%)
  Xerostomia (3%)

OXYCODONE

Trade names: Endocodone; OxyContin (Purdue); OxyIR (Purdue); Percocet (Endo); Roxicodone (aaiPharma); Tylox (Ortho-McNeil)
Other common trade name: *Supeudol*
Indications: Pain
Category: Narcotic analgesic
Half-life: 4.6 hours
Clinically important, potentially hazardous interactions with: cimetidine, clonazepam

Oxycodone is often combined with acetaminophen (Percocet, Roxicet, Tylox) or aspirin (Percodan, Roxiprin)

Reactions

Skin
Baboon syndrome [1]
Diaphoresis
Pruritus [3]
Rash (sic) (<1%)
Urticaria (<1%)

Other
Death [1]
Headache
Injection-site pain (1–10%)
Xerostomia (1–10%)

PANCURONIUM

Other common trade names: *Alpax; Bromurex; Curon-B; Panconium; Pansian*
Indications: Anesthesia adjunct, neuromuscular blockade, muscle relaxant
Category: Nondepolarizing neuromuscular blockade
Half-life: 89–161 minutes
Clinically important, potentially hazardous interactions with: aminoglycosides, cyclopropane, enflurane, gentamicin, halothane, isoflurane, kanamycin, methoxyflurane, neomycin, piperacillin, streptomycin, tobramycin

Reactions

Skin
Burning
Edema
Erythema [1]
Pruritus
Rash (sic)

Cardiovascular
Flushing

Other
Anaphylactoid reactions [9]
Hypersensitivity [1]
Myalgia [3]
Rhabdomyolysis [1]
Sialorrhea

PANTOPRAZOLE

Trade name: Protonix (Wyeth)
Indications: Esophagitis associated with Gastroesophageal Reflux Disease (GERD)
Category: Proton pump (gastric acid secretion) inhibitor
Half-life: 1 hour
Clinically important, potentially hazardous interactions with: eucalyptus

---

Reactions

Skin
  Abscess (<1%)
  Acne (<1%)
  Allergic reactions (sic) (<1%)
  Angioedema (<1%)
  Balanitis (<1%)
  Dermatitis (<1%)
  Diaphoresis (<1%) [1]
  Eczema (<1%)
  Edema (<1%)
  Erythema multiforme (<1%)
  Exanthems (<1%)
  Facial edema (<1%) [1]
  Flu-like syndrome (1–10%)
  Fungal dermatitis (<1%)
  Herpes simplex (<1%)
  Herpes zoster (<1%)
  Infections (1–10%)
  Lichenoid eruption (<1%) [1]
  Lupus erythematosus (discoid) [1]
  Peripheral edema [2]
  Photosensitivity [1]
  Phototoxicity [1]
  Pruritus (<1%) [1]
  Rash (sic) (<1%) [2]
  Stevens–Johnson syndrome (<1%)
  Toxic epidermal necrolysis (<1%)
  Ulcerations (<1%)
  Urticaria (<1%) [2]
  Xerosis (<1%)

Hair
  Hair – alopecia (<1%)

Hematopoietic
  Ecchymoses (<1%)

Other
  Anaphylactoid reactions (<1%) [4]
  Aphthous stomatitis (<1%)
  Arthralgia [1]
  Dysgeusia (<1%)
  Fatigue [1]
  Fever [1]
  Foetor ex ore (halitosis) (<1%)
  Gingivitis (<1%)
  Glossitis (<1%)
  Headache
  Hyperesthesia (<1%)
  Hypersensitivity [1]
  Mastodynia (<1%)
  Myalgia (<1%)
  Oral candidiasis (<1%)
  Paresthesias (<1%)
  Sialorrhea (<1%)
  Stomatitis (<1%)
  Thrombophlebitis (<1%)
  Tongue edema [1]
  Tongue pigmentation (<1%)
  Tremor (<1%)
  Vaginitis (<1%)
  Xerostomia (<1%)

PAPAVERINE

Trade names: Genabid; Pavabid; Pavatine
Other common trade names: *Angioverin; Optenyl; Pameion; Papaverine 60; Papaverini; Pavagen; Pavased*
Indications: Peripheral and cerebral ischemia
Category: Peripheral vasodilator
Half-life: 0.5–2 hours

Reactions

Skin
  Diaphoresis (<1%)
  Exanthems
  Fixed eruption [1]
  Pruritus (<1%)
  Pyogenic granuloma [1]
  Rash (sic)
  Toxic epidermal necrolysis [1]
  Urticaria

Cardiovascular
  Flushing (<1%)

Other
  Headache
  Injection-site thrombophlebitis (<1%)
  Priapism (11%) [3]
  Xerostomia (<1%)

PARAMETHADIONE

Indications: Absence (petit-mal) seizures
Category: Anticonvulsant
Half-life: 12–24 hours

Reactions

Skin
  Acne
  Erythema multiforme [2]
  Exanthems
  Exfoliative dermatitis [1]
  Lupus erythematosus
  Pruritus

Hair
  Hair – alopecia

Other
  Gingivitis
  Oral mucosal eruption [1]
  Paresthesias

PEMOLINE

Trade name: Cylert (Abbott)
Other common trade names: *Betanamin; Tradon*
Indications: Attention deficit disorder, narcolepsy
Category: Anorexiant; Central nervous system stimulant
Half-life: 9–14 hours
Clinically important, potentially hazardous interactions with: pimozide

Reactions

Skin
  Exanthems (<1%) [1]
  Rash (sic) (>10%)

Other
  Headache

Parkinsonism
Rhabdomyolysis [1]
Tourette's syndrome

PENICILLAMINE

Trade name: Depen (MedPointe)
Other common trade names: *Artamin; D-Penamine; Distamine; Kelatin; Pendramine*
Indications: Wilson's disease, rheumatoid arthritis
Category: Antidote; Chelating agent
Half-life: 1.7–3.2 hours
Clinically important, potentially hazardous interactions with: aluminum hydroxide, antacids, ascorbic acid, bone marrow suppressants, chloroquine, cytotoxic agents, food, gold, hydroxychloroquine, iron, magnesium, primaquine, probenecid

Note: For excellent reviews of many of the cutaneous manifestations caused by penicillamine see (1983): Levy RS+, *J Am Acad Dermatol* 8, 548 and (1981): Sternlieb I+, *J Rheumatol* 8 (Suppl 7), 149

Reactions

Skin
  Anetoderma [1]
  Atrophy [1]
  Bullous eruption [3]
  Bullous pemphigoid [5]
  Cutis laxa [8]
  Cyst [1]
  Dermatitis [2]
  Dermatomyositis [12]
  Dermopathy [1]
  Edema of lip (1–10%) [1]
  Ehlers–Danlos syndrome [2]

Elastosis perforans serpiginosa [25]
Epidermolysis bullosa [3]
Epidermolysis bullosa acquisita [1]
Erythema multiforme (1–5%)
Erythema nodosum (<1%) [1]
Exanthems [7]
Exfoliative dermatitis
Facial edema [1]
Fragility [1]
Graft-versus-host reaction [1]
Lathyrism [1]
Lichen planus [4]

Lichenoid eruption [7]
Lupus erythematosus [40]
Morphea [2]
Papular lesions at site of trauma [1]
Pemphigus [63]
Pemphigus erythematodes (Senear–Usher) [9]
Pemphigus foliaceus [16]
Pemphigus herpetiformis [3]
Pemphigus vulgaris [1]
Peripheral edema (1–10%)
Pruritus (44–50%) [2]
Pseudoxanthoma elasticum [11]
Psoriasis [4]
Purpura [4]
Rash (sic) (44–50%) [5]
Scleroderma [3]
Sjøgren's syndrome [1]
Stevens–Johnson syndrome [1]
Toxic epidermal necrolysis (<1%) [2]
Urticaria (44–50%) [2]
Vasculitis [6]
Vesiculation [1]
Wrinkling (sic) [1]
Xerosis [1]

Hair
Hair – alopecia [2]
Hair – hirsutism [2]

Nails
Nails – dystrophy [1]
Nails – elkonyxis (punched-out appearance of the nail at lunulae) [1]
Nails – leukonychia [1]
Nails – longitudinal ridges [1]
Nails – onychoschizia [1]
Nails – pigmentation [4]

Hematopoietic
Ecchymoses

Cardiovascular
Flushing [1]

Other
Ageusia (12%) [2]
Aphthous stomatitis [1]
Bromhidrosis [1]
Cicatricial pemphigoid [2]
Death
Dysgeusia (metallic taste) [4]
Gingivitis
Glossitis [1]
Guillain–Barré syndrome [1]
Gynecomastia [3]
Hypersensitivity [2]
Hypogeusia (25–33%) [2]
Mucocutaneous reactions (sic) [1]
Mucosal lesions (pemphigus-like) [2]
Mucosal ulceration [1]
Oral lichenoid eruption [1]
Oral ulceration [5]
Polymyositis [3]
Serum sickness [1]
Stomatitis [5]
Tinnitus

PENTAZOCINE

Trade name: Talwin (Hospira)
Other common trade names: *Fortral; Fortwin; Liticon; Ospronim; Pentafen; Sosegon; Susevin; Talacen*
Indications: Pain
Category: Narcotic; Opioid analgesic; Sedative
Half-life: 2–3 hours
Clinically important, potentially hazardous interactions with: cimetidine, morphine

Reactions

Skin
Cellulitis [1]
Dermatitis
Diaphoresis
Exanthems [1]
Facial edema
Generalized eruption (sic) [1]
Pigmentation (surrounding ulcers) [1]
Pruritus (<1%)
Rash (sic) (1–10%)
Scleroderma [2]
Sclerosis [3]
Toxic epidermal necrolysis (<1%) [2]
Ulcerations [6]
Urticaria

Cardiovascular
Flushing [1]

Other
Dysgeusia

Embolia cutis medicamentosa (Nicolau
   syndrome) [1]
Fibromyalgia [2]
Injection-site calcification [2]
Injection-site fibrosis [1]
Injection-site granuloma [3]
Injection-site induration [9]
Injection-site pain
Injection-site pigmentation [1]
Lipogranulomas [1]
Myofibrosis [1]
Panniculitis (chronic) [1]
Paresthesias
Phlebitis [1]
Soft tissue calcification [1]
Tinnitus
Xerostomia (1–10%)

PENTOBARBITAL

Other common trade names: *Medinox Mono; Mintal; Nova Rectal; Pentobarbitone; Prodromol; Sombutol*
Indications: Insomnia, sedation
Category: Anticonvulsant; Barbiturate sedative-hypnotic
Half-life: 15–50 hours
Clinically important, potentially hazardous interactions with: alcohol, anticoagulants, antihistamines, brompheniramine, buclizine, chlorpheniramine, dicumarol, ethanolamine, imatinib, nalbuphine, warfarin

Reactions

Skin
Acne
Angioedema (<1%)
Bullous eruption [1]
Erythema multiforme [1]
Exanthems [1]
Exfoliative dermatitis (<1%) [1]
Fixed eruption [1]

Herpes simplex (activation)
Lupus erythematosus [2]
Necrosis [1]
Photosensitivity [1]
Pruritus
Purpura [1]
Rash (sic) (<1%)
Stevens–Johnson syndrome (<1%)

Toxic epidermal necrolysis [1]
Urticaria
Vasculitis

Other
Headache
Hypersensitivity

Injection-site pain (1–10%)
Injection-site reactions (sic) (<1%)
Oral ulceration
Porphyria [1]
Porphyria variegata
Rhabdomyolysis [1]
Thrombophlebitis (<1%)

PENTOSAN

Synonym: PPS
Trade name: Elmiron (Ortho-McNeil)
Indications: Bladder pain, interstitial cystitis
Category: Urinary analgesic
Half-life: 4.8 hours

Reactions

Skin
Allergic reactions (sic) (<1%)
Photosensitivity (<1%)
Pruritus (<1%)
Purpura (<1%)
Rash (sic) (1–10%)
Urticaria (<1%)

Hair
Hair – alopecia (1–10%)

Hematopoietic
Ecchymoses

Other
Gingivitis (<1%)
Headache
Oral ulceration (<1%)

PEPPERMINT

Scientific name: *Mentha piperita*
Family: Labiatae
Trade and other common names: Aludrox; brandy mint; Colpermin; Enteroplant (peppermint and caraway oils); menthol; PCC
Category: Analgesic; Antiemetic; Antiseptic; Carminative; Cholagogue; Choleretic; Diaphoretic; Disinfectant; Peripheral vasodilator; Spasmolytic
Purported indications and other uses: Dyspepsia, regress pancreatic, mammary, and liver tumors, irritable bowel syndrome, colonic spasm, colic, nausea, vomiting, biliary disorders, common cold, dysmenorrhoea, anxiolytic. **Topical:** pain, itching, inflammations, headaches, toothache, pruritus, urticaria, mosquito repellant. **Vapor:** bronchial catarrh, fever, influenza. Flavoring, cosmetics, toothpaste, mouthwash
Half-life: N/A
Clinically important, potentially hazardous interactions with: cisapride

Reactions

Skin
Adverse effects (sic) [2]
Allergic reactions (sic) [1]
Burning (anal) [1]
Cheilitis [2]
Dermatitis [3]
Lichenoid eruption [1]
Perioral dermatitis [1]
Rash (sic) [1]
Sensitivity [2]

Other
Burning mouth syndrome [1]
Gingivitis [1]
Glossitis [1]
Hypersensitivity [2]
Oral ulceration [2]
Side effects (sic) [2]
Stomatitis [2]
Toxicity [1]

PERGOLIDE

Trade name: Permax (Lilly)
Other common trade names: *Celance; Parkotil; Pergolide*
Indications: Parkinsonism
Category: Antiparkinsonian; Dopamine receptor agonist; Ergot alkaloid
Half-life: 27 hours

Reactions

Skin
Acne
Chills (1–10%)
Diaphoresis (2.1%)
Discoloration
Edema (1.6%)
Exanthems
Facial edema (1.1%) [1]
Flu-like syndrome (1–10%)
Neuroleptic malignant syndrome [1]
Peripheral edema (1–10%)
Pruritus
Rash (sic) (3.2%)
Seborrhea
Ulcerations
Urticaria
Vasculitis [2]

Xerosis

Hair
Hair – alopecia
Hair – hirsutism

Other
Dysgeusia (1.6%)
Erythromelalgia [2]
Gingivitis (<1%)
Mastodynia
Myalgia (<1%)
Paresthesias (1.6%)
Priapism
Tinnitus
Tremor (1–10%)
Xerostomia (1–10%)

PHELLODENDRON

Scientific names: *Phellodendron amurense; Phellodendron chinense; Phellodendron wilsonii*
Family: Rutaceae
Trade and other common names: Amur Cork-tree; Chuan huangbo; Cortex Phellodendri; Guan huangbo; Huang Bai; Nexrutine (Next Pharma); phellamurin. Ingredient in Oren-gedoku-to, zhi bai kuncao tang and Shangke Wangshui
Category: Antioxidant; Bactericide; COX-2 inhibitor; Immunosuppressant
Purported indications and other uses: anti-inflammatory, muscle and joint pain, gastroenteritis, abdominal pain, diarrhea, gastric ulcers, thrush, cholera, night sweats, fever, nocturnal emissions, dysentery, jaundice, leukorrhea, weakness and edema of legs, consumptive fever. **Topical:** sores, sores, skin infection with local redness and swelling, eczema with itching, periodontal disease (in dentifrice)
Half-life: N/A
Clinically important, potentially hazardous interactions with: aspirin, cyclosporine, NSAIDs

Reactions

Skin   Edema
  Bleeding
Note: Should not be taken with impaired renal function, heart function, or hypertension

PHENAZOPYRIDINE

Trade names: Baridium; Geridium; Prodium; Pyridiate; Pyridium (Warner Chilcott)
Other common trade names: *Azodine; Eridium; Phenazo; Pyronium; Sedural; Urodine; Urogesic; Urohman; Uropyridin*
Indications: Urinary urgency, dysuria
Category: Urinary analgesic
Half-life: N/A

Reactions

Skin
  Allergic reactions (sic) (<1%) [1]
  Edema
  Exanthems (<1%) [1]
  Pigmentation (<1%) [2]
  Pruritus
  Rash (sic) (<1%)

Nails
  Nails – pigmentation [1]

Other
  Anaphylactoid reactions
  Headache

PHENOBARBITAL

Synonyms: phenobarbitone; phenylethylmalonylurea
Trade names: Barbita; Luminal (Sanofi-Aventis); Solfoton
Other common trade names: *Alepsal; Barbilixir; Barbital; Gardenal; Luminaletten; Phenaemal; Phenobarbitone*
Indications: Insomnia, seizures
Category: Barbiturate sedative-hypnotic
Half-life: 2–6 days
Clinically important, potentially hazardous interactions with: alcohol, anticoagulants, antihistamines, brompheniramine, buclizine, chlorpheniramine, delavirdine, dicumarol, ethanolamine, fluconazole, fosamprenavir, imatinib, influenza vaccines, meperidine, midazolam, solifenacin, telithromycin, warfarin

---

Reactions

Skin
  Acne [1]
  Acute generalized exanthematous
    pustulosis (AGEP) [1]
  Allergic reactions (sic) [2]
  Angioedema (<1%)
  Anticonvulsant hypersensitivity syndrome
    [3]
  Bullous eruption [5]
  Depigmentation [1]
  Edema
  Erythema multiforme [7]
  Erythroderma [1]
  Exanthems [10]
  Exfoliative dermatitis (<1%) [6]
  Fixed eruption [7]
  Graft-versus-host reaction [1]
  Herpes simplex (activation)
  Lupus erythematosus [2]
  Necrosis [1]
  Pemphigus [1]
  Peripheral edema [1]
  Photosensitivity [1]
  Pruritus [1]
  Purpura [2]
  Pustules (generalized) [1]
  Rash (sic) (<1%)
  Stevens–Johnson syndrome (<1%) [12]

  Toxic epidermal necrolysis [19]
  Toxicoderma [1]
  Urticaria [1]
  Vasculitis

Hair
  Hair – depigmentation [1]

Nails
  Nails – hypoplasia [2]

Other
  Acute intermittent porphyria [1]
  Death
  DRESS syndrome [4]
  Gingival hypertrophy [1]
  Headache
  Hypersensitivity (<1%) [7]
  Hypoplasia of phalanges [2]
  Injection-site bullous eruption [1]
  Injection-site pain (>10%)
  Injection-site thrombophlebitis (>10%)
  Oral ulceration
  Osteomalacia [1]
  Porphyria cutanea tarda [1]
  Porphyria variegata
  Rhabdomyolysis [1]
  Xerostomia [1]

PHENSUXIMIDE

Indications: Petit mal seizures
Category: Anticonvulsant
Half-life: 5–12 hours

Reactions

Skin
  Erythema multiforme (<1%)
  Lupus erythematosus
  Pruritus
  Purpura [1]
  Rash (sic)
  Stevens–Johnson syndrome

Hair
  Hair – alopecia

Hair – hirsutism

Eyes
  Periorbital edema

Other
  Acute intermittent porphyria
  Gingival hypertrophy
  Oral ulceration

PHENYTOIN

Synonyms: diphenylhydantoin; DPH; phenytoin sodium
Trade names: Dilantin (Pfizer); Phenytek (Mylan Bertek)
Other common trade names: *Di-Hydran; Diphenylan; Epanutin; Fenytoin; Phenhydan; Pyoredol; Zentropil*
Indications: Grand mal seizures
Category: Antiarrhythmic; Hydantoin anticonvulsant
Half-life: 7–42 hours (dose dependent)
Clinically important, potentially hazardous interactions with: amprenavir, aprepitant, calcium, chloramphenicol, cimetidine, clorazepate, cyclosporine, delavirdine, diazoxide, disulfiram, dopamine, fluconazole, fluoxetine, fosamprenavir, ginkgo biloba, imatinib, indinavir, influenza vaccines, isoniazid, isradipine, itraconazole, meperidine, midazolam, nelfinavir, primrose, ritonavir, sage, saquinavir, solifenacin, st john's wort, sucralfate, telithromycin, ticlopidine, vigabatrin

An excellent overview of cutaneous reactions to phenytoin can be found in (1988): Silverman AK+, *J Am Acad Dermatol* 18, 721

Note: About 19% of patients receiving phenytoin develop skin reactions (1983): Rapp RP+, *Neurosurg* 13, 272. They typically develop 10 to 14 days following the start of treatment

Reactions

Skin
  Acne [7]
  Acute generalized exanthematous
    pustulosis (AGEP) [2]

Angioedema [2]
Anticonvulsant hypersensitivity syndrome
  [2]
Bullous eruption [1]

Dermatomyositis [1]
Eosinophilic fasciitis [1]
Epidermolysis bullosa [1]
Erythema multiforme [11]
Erythroderma [4]
Exanthems (6–71%) [15]
Exfoliative dermatitis [12]
Fixed eruption [3]
Heel pad thickening [1]
Lichen planus [1]
Lichenoid eruption [1]
Linear IgA dermatosis [5]
Lupus erythematosus [16]
Lymphoma (<1%) [5]
Mucocutaneous lymph node syndrome
  (Kawasaki syndrome) [1]
Mycosis fungoides [4]
Necrosis [1]
Pemphigus [1]
Peripheral edema [1]
Pigmentation [1]
Pruritus [6]
Pseudoacanthosis nigricans [1]
Purple glove syndrome [5]
Purpura [4]
Pustules [3]
Rash (sic) (1–10%) [3]
Reticular hyperplasia [2]
Rhinophyma [1]
Scleroderma [1]
Sezary syndrome [1]
Sjøgren's syndrome [1]
Stevens–Johnson syndrome (14%) [27]
Toxic dermatitis [1]
Toxic epidermal necrolysis (2%) [39]
Urticaria [4]
Vasculitis (2%) [6]
Warts [1]

Hair
Hair – alopecia [3]
Hair – hirsutism [5]
Hair – hypertrichosis [2]

Nails
Nails – changes (sic) [2]
Nails – hypoplasia [3]
Nails – onychopathy [1]
Nails – pigmentation [1]

Cardiovascular
Arrhythmias [1]
Bradycardia [1]
Congestive heart failure [1]

Other
Acromegaloid features [1]
Acute intermittent porphyria [1]
Ageusia [2]
Application-site pain [1]
Coarse facies [2]
Death
Digital malformations [3]
Dyskinesia [2]
Fetal hydantoin syndrome* [7]
Gingival hypertrophy (>10%) [27]
Gynecomastia [1]
Headache
Hypersensitivity** [32]
Injection-site extravasation [1]
Injection-site necrosis [2]
Injection-site pain [1]
Lymphadenopathy [1]
Lymphoproliferative disease [1]
Mucocutaneous eruption [2]
Myalgia [2]
Oral ulceration [1]
Osteomalacia [1]
Paresthesias (<1%) [2]
Periarteritis nodosa [2]
Peyronie's disease
Polyfibromatosis [1]
Polymyositis [1]
Porphyria [1]
Porphyria cutanea tarda [1]
Pseudolymphoma (<1%) [29]
Rhabdomyolysis [2]
Serum sickness [2]
Thrombophlebitis (<1%)

*Note: The fetal hydantoin syndrome (FHS) – children whose mothers receive phenytoin during pregnancy are born with FHS. The main features of this syndrome are mental and growth retardation, unusual facies, digital and nail hypoplasia, and coarse scalp hair. Occasionally neonatal acne will be present

PHYSOSTIGMINE

Synonyms: Eserine salicylates; Physostigmine salicylates; Physostigmine sulfate
Trade names: Antilirium; Isopto Eserine
Indications: Miotic in glaucoma treatment, reverses toxic CNS effects caused by anticholinergic drugs
Category: Anticholinesterase; Antidote; Antiglaucoma
Half-life: 15–40 minutes
Clinically important, potentially hazardous interactions with: bethanechol, corticosteroids, galantamine, methacholine, succinylcholine

Reactions

Skin
  Diaphoresis (>10%)
  Erythema (1–10%) [1]

Eyes
  Lacrimation (>10%)
  Ocular burning (1–10%)
  Ocular stinging (>10%)

Cardiovascular
  Atrial fibrillation [1]
  Bradycardia [2]
  Tachycardia [1]

Other
  Death
  Seizures (1–10%) [3]
  Sialorrhea (>10%)
  Twitching (1–10%)

Note: Antilirium is a derivative of the Calabar bean, and its active moiety, physostigmine, is also known as eserine.
Note: Physostigmine is used to reverse the effect upon the nervous system caused by clinical or toxic dosages of drugs and herbs capable of producing the Anticholinergic syndrome.
Some of the drugs responsible are: amitriptyline, amoxapine, atropine, benztropine, biperiden, clidinium, cyclobenzaprine, desipramine, doxepin, hyoscyamine, imipramine, lorazepam, maprotiline, nortriptyline, protriptyline, propantheline, scopolamine, trimipramine. Some herbals that can elicit the anticholinergic syndrome are black henbane, deadly nightshade, Devil's apple, Jimson weed, Loco seeds or weeds, Matrimony vine, night blooming jessamine, stinkweed.

PIPECURONIUM

Indications: Adjunct to general anesthesia
Category: Nondepolarizing neuromuscular blocking agent
Half-life: 2–3 hours
Clinically important, potentially hazardous interactions with: anesthetics (inhalational), antibiotics, gentamicin, magnesium salts, quinidine, succinylcholine

Reactions

Skin
  Rash (sic) (<1%)
  Urticaria (<1%)

Other
  Hyperesthesia (<1%)
  Muscle atrophy (<1%)

PIROXICAM

Trade name: Feldene (Pfizer)
Other common trade names: *Antiflog; Apo-Piroxicam; Baxo; Doblexan; Felden; Larapam; Nu-Pirox; Rogal; Sotilen; Zunden*
Indications: Arthritis
Category: Analgesic; Nonsteroidal anti-inflammatory (NSAID)
Half-life: 50 hours
Clinically important, potentially hazardous interactions with: methotrexate, ritonavir

Reactions

Skin
  Allergic reactions (sic) [1]
  Angioedema (<1%) [1]
  Bullous dermatitis [1]
  Dermatitis [5]
  Diaphoresis (<1%) [1]
  Dyshidrosis [1]
  Edema (>1%)
  Erythema (<1%)
  Erythema annulare centrifugum [1]
  Erythema multiforme (<1%) [12]
  Erythroderma [2]
  Exanthems (>5%) [9]
  Exfoliative dermatitis (<1%) [1]
  Fixed eruption [10]
  Lichenoid eruption [5]
  Linear IgA dermatosis [3]
  Lupus erythematosus [1]
  Pemphigus [2]
  Pemphigus foliaceus [1]
  Peripheral edema [1]
  Petechiae (<1%)
  Photosensitivity (<1%) [39]
  Pruritus (1–10%) [5]
  Purpura (<1%) [2]
  Rash (sic) (>10%)
  Side effects (sic) (46.9%) [1]
  Stevens–Johnson syndrome (<1%) [2]
  Toxic dermatitis [1]
  Toxic epidermal necrolysis (<1%) [12]
  Urticaria (<1%) [5]
  Vasculitis (<1%) [3]
  Vesiculation (<1%) [2]

Hair
  Hair – alopecia [3]

Nails
  Nails – onycholysis

Hematopoietic
  Ecchymoses (<1%)

Cardiovascular
  Hot flashes (<1%)

Other
  Anaphylactoid reactions (<1%)
  Aphthous stomatitis [3]

Death [1]
Fixed intraoral eruption [1]
Headache
Oral ulceration [1]
Paresthesias [1]
Pseudoporphyria [1]
Serum sickness (<1%)
Stomatitis (>1%)
Tinnitus
Xerostomia (<1%)

PRAMIPEXOLE

Trade name: Mirapex (Pfizer) (Boehringer Ingelheim)
Indications: Parkinsonism
Category: Antiparkinsonian
Half-life: ~8 hours

Reactions

Skin
  Adverse effects (sic) (2%)
  Allergic reactions (sic) (>1%)
  Diaphoresis (>1%)
  Edema (5%)
  Peripheral edema (5%) [1]
  Pruritus (>1%)
  Rash (sic) (>1%)

Other
  Dysgeusia (>1%)

Headache
Hyperesthesia (3%)
Myalgia (>1%)
Paresthesias (>1%)
Sialorrhea (>1%)
Tooth disorder (>1%)
Twitching (2%)
Xerostomia (7%) [1]

PRIMIDONE

Trade name: Mysoline (Xcel)
Other common trade names: *Midone; Mylepsin; PMS Primidone; Prysoline; Sertan*
Indications: Seizures
Category: Anticonvulsant; Barbiturate
Half-life: 10–12 hours
Clinically important, potentially hazardous interactions with: alcohol, anticoagulants, antihistamines, brompheniramine, buclizine, chlorpheniramine, dicumarol, ethanolamine*, imatinib, midazolam, niacinamide, warfarin

Reactions

Skin
  Acne
  Allergic reactions (sic) [1]
  Erythema multiforme (<1%) [3]
  Exanthems (1–5%) [1]
  Exfoliative dermatitis
  Lupus erythematosus (<1%) [6]
  Rash (sic) (<1%)
  Toxic epidermal necrolysis [4]

  Urticaria [1]

Other
  Acute intermittent porphyria
  Gingival hypertrophy
  Hypersensitivity* [2]
  Mucocutaneous syndrome [1]
  Osteomalacia [1]
  Rhabdomyolysis [1]

PROCYCLIDINE

Trade name: Kemadrin (Monarch)
Other common trade names: *Apricolin; Kemadren; Onservan; Procyclid*
Indications: Parkinsonism
Category: Anticholinergic; Antidyskinetic; Antiparkinsonian
Duration of action: 4 hours
Clinically important, potentially hazardous interactions with: anticholinergics, arbutamine

Reactions

Skin
  Hypohidrosis (>10%)
  Photosensitivity (1–10%)
  Rash (sic) (<1%)
  Urticaria

  Xerosis (>10%)

Other
  Xerostomia (>10%)

PROPANTHELINE

Trade name: Propantheline
Other common trade names: *Bropantil; Corrigast; Ercoril; Ercotina; Norproban; Propantel*
Indications: Peptic ulcer
Category: Antispasmodic; Gastrointestinal anticholinergic
Half-life: 1.6 hours
Clinically important, potentially hazardous interactions with: anticholinergics, arbutamine, digoxin

Reactions

Skin
  Allergic reactions (sic)
  Dermatitis [6]
  Diaphoresis (>10%)

  Exanthems
  Hypohidrosis
  Rash (sic) (<1%)
  Urticaria

Xerosis (>10%)

Other
Ageusia
Anaphylactoid reactions

Dysgeusia
Headache
Sialopenia
Xerostomia (>10%)

PROPOFOL

Trade name: Diprivan (AstraZeneca)
Indications: Induction and maintenance of anesthesia
Category: General anesthetic; Sedative
Half-life: initial: 40 minutes; terminal: 3 days
Clinically important, potentially hazardous interactions with: telithromycin

Reactions

Skin
Allergic reactions (sic) [1]
Edema (<1%)
Exanthems (6%) [2]
Fixed eruption (1%)
Pruritus (>1%) [1]
Rash (sic) (5%)
Raynaud's phenomenon [1]
Urticaria [2]

Hair
Hair – pigmentation [2]

Cardiovascular
Bradycardia [4]
Flushing (>1%)

Other
Anaphylactoid reactions (1–10%) [6]
Cough [2]
Death [4]
Dysgeusia (<1%)
Injection-site erythema (<1%)
Injection-site pain (>10%) [26]
Injection-site pruritus (<1%)
Myalgia (>1%)
Phlebitis
Rhabdomyolysis [2]
Seizures [1]
Sialorrhea (>1%)
Tinnitus
Twitching (1–10%)
Xerostomia (<1%)

PROPOXYPHENE

Trade names: Darvocet-N (aaiPharma); Darvon (Lilly); Darvon Compound (aaiPharma)
Other common trade names: *Algafan; Antalvic; Develin; Dolotard; Doloxene; Liberan; Parvon*
Indications: Pain
Category: Narcotic analgesic
Half-life: 8–24 hours

Clinically important, potentially hazardous interactions with: alcohol, alprazolam, ritonavir, warfarin

Darvocet is propoxyphene and acetaminophen; Darvon Compound is propoxyphene and aspirin

Reactions

Skin
  Diaphoresis
  Exanthems [1]
  Facial edema
  Pruritus
  Rash (sic) (<1%)
  Urticaria (<1%)

Cardiovascular
  Flushing

Other
  Anal ulceration [1]
  Injection-site nodules [1]
  Injection-site pain (1–10%)
  Trembling
  Xerostomia (1–10%)

PROPRANOLOL

Trade names: Inderal (Wyeth); Inderide (Wyeth)
Other common trade names: *Acifol; Apsolol; Betabloc; Cinlol; Detensol; Inderalici; Inderex; Novo-Pranol; Prosin; Sinal; Tesnol*
Indications: Hypertension, angina pectoris
Category: Antianginal; Antiarrhythmic class II; Antihypertensive; Beta-adrenoceptor blocker
Half-life: 2–6 hours
Clinically important, potentially hazardous interactions with: cimetidine, clonidine, epinephrine, eucalyptus, haloperidol, insulin, insulin glargine, terbutaline, verapamil

Inderide is propranolol and hydrochlorothiazide

Note: Cutaneous side effects of beta-receptor blockaders are clinically polymorphous. They apparently appear after several months of continuous therapy. Atypical psoriasiform, lichen planus-like, and eczematous chronic rashes are mainly observed. (1983): Hödl St, *Z Hautkr* (German) 58, 17

Reactions

Skin
  Acne [1]
  Angioedema [1]
  Bullous eruption [1]
  Cheilitis [1]
  Dermatitis [2]
  Diaphoresis
  Eczema [2]
  Edema
  Erythema (systemic) [1]
  Erythema multiforme [1]
  Exanthems (<1%) [5]
  Exfoliative dermatitis [1]
  Hyperkeratosis (palms and soles)

Lichenoid eruption [3]
Lupus erythematosus [2]
Necrosis
Pemphigus [2]
Peripheral edema
Peripheral skin necrosis [2]
Photosensitivity [1]
Phototoxicity [1]
Pruritus [2]
Psoriasis [16]
Purpura [1]
Pustular psoriasis [2]
Rash (sic) (1–10%)
Raynaud's phenomenon (59%) [1]

Sclerosis [1]
Stevens–Johnson syndrome [2]
Toxic epidermal necrolysis [1]
Toxicoderma [1]
Urticaria [3]
Xerosis

Hair

Hair – alopecia [6]
Hair – alopecia areata [1]

Nails

Nails – discoloration [1]
Nails – onycholysis [1]
Nails – pitting (psoriasiform) [1]
Nails – thickening [2]

Cardiovascular

Arrhythmias [1]
Bradycardia [9]

Flushing [2]
Hypertension [1]
Hypotension [1]
QT prolongation [1]

Other

Anaphylactoid reactions [1]
Dupuytren's contracture [1]
Dysgeusia [1]
Headache
Myalgia [1]
Oral ulceration [1]
Paresthesias
Peyronie's disease [6]
Serum sickness [1]
Tongue pigmentation [1]
Xerostomia

QUINUPRISTIN/DALFOPRISTIN

Synonyms: pristinamycin; RP59500
Trade name: Synercid (Monarch)
Indications: Serious life-threatening bacterial infections
Category: Streptogramin antibiotic
Half-life: 1.3–1.5 hours

Reactions

Skin

Acute febrile neutrophilic dermatosis
  (Sweet's syndrome) [1]
Allergic reactions (sic) (<1%)
Candidiasis (<1%)
Diaphoresis (<1%)
Exanthems (<1%)
Peripheral edema (<1%)
Pruritus (1.5%)
Rash (sic) (2–4%) [1]
Ulcerations (<1%)
Urticaria (<1%)

Other

Anaphylactoid reactions (<1%)

Arthralgia [5]
Arthralgia [1]
Injection-site edema (17.3%) [1]
Injection-site extravasation (42%) [1]
Injection-site pain (40%) [2]
Injection-site reactions (sic) (13.4%)
Myalgia (<1–5%) [6]
Oral candidiasis (<1%)
Paresthesias (<1%)
Phlebitis (<1%)
Stomatitis (<1%)
Thrombophlebitis (2.4%) [1]
Tremor (<1%)
Vaginitis (<1%)

RABEPRAZOLE

Synonym: pariprazole
Trade name: Aciphex (Eisai) (Janssen)
Indications: Gastroesophageal reflux disease (GERD)
Category: Proton pump (gastric acid secretion) inhibitor
Half-life: 1–2 hours

Reactions

Skin
  Allergic reactions (sic) (<1%)
  Chills (<1%)
  Diaphoresis (<1%)
  Edema
  Facial edema (<1%)
  Herpes zoster (<1%)
  Peripheral edema (<1%)
  Photosensitivity (<1%)
  Pigmentation (<1%)
  Pruritus (<1%)
  Psoriasis (<1%)
  Purpura
  Rash (sic) (<1%)
  Urticaria (<1%)
  Xerosis (<1%)

Hair
  Hair – alopecia (<1%)

Hematopoietic
  Ecchymoses (<1%)

Other
  Gingivitis (<1%)
  Glossitis (<1%)
  Gynecomastia (<1%)
  Headache
  Myalgia (<1%)
  Oral ulceration
  Paresthesias (<1%)
  Rhabdomyolysis [1]
  Stomatitis (<1%) [1]
  Thrombophlebitis (<1%)
  Tongue edema [1]
  Tremor (<1%)
  Twitching (<1%)
  Xerostomia (<1%)

RANITIDINE

Trade name: Zantac (GSK)
Other common trade names: *Apo-Ranitidine; Axoban; Azantac; Nu-Ranit; Raniben; Raniplex; Ranisen; Sostril; Zantab; Zantac-C; Zantic*
Indications: Duodenal ulcer
Category: Antihistamine H_2-blocker ; Antiulcer
Half-life: 2.5 hours
Clinically important, potentially hazardous interactions with: alfentanil, devil's claw, fentanyl

Note: Ranitidine is present in mother's milk in relatively large amounts. It is thought that gynecomastia develops as a result of ranitidine blocking the androgen receptors at the end organs

Reactions

Skin
  Acute generalized exanthematous
    pustulosis (AGEP) [1]
  Angioedema (<1%)
  Dermatitis [5]
  Eczema [2]
  Erythema multiforme
  Exanthems [4]
  Fixed eruption [1]
  Lichenoid eruption [1]
  Lupus erythematosus [1]
  Photosensitivity [2]
  Pruritus (<1%) [1]
  Psoriasis [1]
  Purpura [2]
  Pustules
  Rash (sic) (1–10%) [1]
  Stevens–Johnson syndrome [1]

  Toxic epidermal necrolysis [2]
  Urticaria [4]
  Vasculitis [1]
  Xerosis

Hair
  Hair – alopecia [1]

Other
  Anaphylactoid reactions [3]
  Dysgeusia [1]
  Gynecomastia (>1%) [3]
  Headache
  Hypersensitivity [1]
  Injection-site burning
  Injection-site pain
  Myalgia
  Porphyria [3]
  Pseudolymphoma [2]

RAPACURONIUM

Trade name: Raplon (Organon)
Indications: To facilitate tracheal intubation
Category: Anesthesia adjunct; Nondepolarizing neuromuscular blockade
Half-life: ~22 days
Clinically important, potentially hazardous interactions with: aminoglycosides, cyclopropane, enflurane, halothane, isoflurane, methoxyflurane, piperacillin

Reactions

Skin
  Diaphoresis (~1%)
  Edema
  Erythema [1]
  Exanthems (>1%)
  Peripheral edema (~1%)
  Pruritus
  Purpura (~1%)
  Rash (sic) (~1%)
  Urticaria (~1%)

Cardiovascular
  Flushing

Other
  Hyperesthesia (~1%)
  Injection-site pain (~1%)
  Injection-site reactions (sic) (~1%) [1]
  Myalgia (~1%)
  Sialorrhea (~1%) [1]
  Thrombophlebitis (~1%)
  Tooth disorder (sic) (~1%)

RED CLOVER

Scientific name: *Trifolium pratense*
Family: Leguminosae
Trade and other common names: Coumestrol; Cow Clover; Cowgrass; Meadow Clover; Menoflavon (Pascoe); Pavine Clover; Promensil (Novogen); Purple Clover; Three-Leaved Grass
Category: Phytoestrogen
Purported indications and other uses: Menopausal symptoms, hot flashes, muscle spasms, hypercholesterolemia, breast pain, osteoporosis, diuretic, expectorant, mild antispasmodic, sedative, blood purifier, bladder infections, liver disorders. Ointment for acne, eczema, psoriasis and other rashes
Half-life: N/A
Clinically important, potentially hazardous interactions with: conjugated estrogens, heparin, ticlopidine, warfarin

Note: Red clover contains phytoestrogens that bind to estrogen and progesterone receptors, potentially adversely affecting breast tissue

Reactions

None

RESVERATROL

Scientific names: *3,4',5-trihydroxystilbene; trans-resveratrol-3-O-glucuronide; trans-resveratrol-3-sulfate*

Family: N/A

Trade and other common names: Kojo-kon; Protykin Resveratrol (Natrol); Resveratrol Antioxidant Protection (Source Naturals)

Category: Anti-inflammatory; antibiotic; antioxidant; antithrombotic; antiviral; cardioprotective; chemopreventive; immunomodulator; neuroprotective; phytoestrogenic

Purported indications and other uses: Cancers, dermal wound healing, atherosclerosis, herpes simplex, cholesterol-lowering, heart disease, skin cancers

Half-life: N/A

Clinically important, potentially hazardous interactions with: aspirin, coumadin

---

Reactions

Skin
  Dermatitis [1]

Note: Resveratrol is extracted from: *Vitis vinifera* – grape seed and skin-, *Polygonium cuspidatum*, and nuts.

Red wine is associated with the so-called French paradox – low incidence of heart disease among French people who drink moderate quantities of red wine but eat a relatively high-fat diet. A glass of red wine contains approximately 640 micrograms of resveratrol

RETEPLASE

Synonyms: recombinant plasminogen activator; r-PA

Trade name: Retavase (Centocor)

Indications: Acute myocardial infarction

Category: Thrombolytic ; Tissue plasminogen activator

Half-life: 13–16 minutes

Clinically important, potentially hazardous interactions with: abciximab, aspirin, bivalirudin, dipyridamole, piperacillin, salicylates

---

Reactions

Skin
  Allergic reactions (sic) (<1%)
  Bleeding
  Purpura

Hematopoietic
  Ecchymoses

Other
  Anaphylactoid reactions (<1%)
  Headache
  Injection-site bleeding (1–10%)

RILUZOLE

Trade name: Rilutek (Sanofi-Aventis)
Indications: Amyotrophic lateral sclerosis (ALS)
Category: Amyotrophic lateral sclerosis (ALS) agent
Half-life: N/A

Reactions

Skin
  Candidiasis
  Cellulitis
  Chills
  Eczema (1.6%)
  Edema
  Exfoliative dermatitis
  Facial edema
  Granulomas
  Peripheral edema (3%)
  Petechiae
  Photosensitivity
  Pruritus
  Purpura

Hair
  Hair – alopecia (1%)

Other
  Abdominal pain (2%) [2]
  Asthenia (5%) [11]

Dizziness [5]
Dysgeusia
Dysphagia [1]
Gingival hemorrhage
Glossitis
Headache [1]
Hyperesthesia
Injection-site reactions (sic)
Mastodynia
Oral candidiasis (0.6%)
Paresthesias (circumoral) [3]
Phlebitis (1%)
Pneumonia (2%) [1]
Stomatitis (1%)
Tongue pigmentation
Tooth disorder (sic) (1%)
Vulvovaginal candidiasis
Xerostomia (3.5%)

RIZATRIPTAN

Synonym: MK462
Trade name: Maxalt (Merck)
Indications: Migraine
Category: Antimigraine; Serotonin agonist
Half-life: 2–3 hours
Clinically important, potentially hazardous interactions with: dihydroergotamine, ergot-containing drugs, isocarboxazid, MAO inhibitors, methysergide, naratriptan, phenelzine, sibutramine, st john's wort, sumatriptan, tranylcypromine, zolmitriptan

Reactions

Skin
  Chills (<1%)

Diaphoresis (<1%)
Facial edema (<1%)

Pruritus (<1%)

Cardiovascular
 Flushing (1–10%)
 Hot flashes (1–10%)

Other
 Dizziness [1]

Headache
Hyperesthesia
Myalgia (<1%)
Paresthesias
Tongue edema
Xerostomia (<5%)

ROFECOXIB*

Trade name: Vioxx (Merck)
Indications: Osteoarthritis, acute pain
Category: Nonsteroidal anti-inflammatory (Cox-2 inhibitor) analgesic
Half-life: 17 hours
Clinically important, potentially hazardous interactions with: anisindione, anticoagulants, dicumarol, lithium, methotrexate, warfarin

*Note: This drug has been withdrawn

Reactions

Skin
 Abrasion (<2%)
 Allergic reactions (sic) (<2%)
 Angioedema [3]
 Atopic dermatitis (<2%)
 Basal cell carcinoma (<2%)
 Bullous eruption (<2%)
 Cellulitis (<2%)
 Dermatitis (<2%)
 Diaphoresis (<2%)
 Edema (3.7%) [2]
 Erythema (<2%) [1]
 Exanthems [1]
 Fixed eruption [3]
 Flu-like syndrome (2.9%)
 Fungal dermatitis (<2%)
 Granuloma annulare [1]
 Herpes simplex (<2%)
 Herpes zoster (<2%)
 Neutrophilic dermatosis [1]
 Nodular eruption [1]
 Peripheral edema (6%) [3]
 Photosensitivity [3]
 Phototoxicity [1]

 Pruritus (<2%) [1]
 Psoriasis [1]
 Purpura [2]
 Rash (sic) (<2%)
 Ulcerations of legs [1]
 Urticaria (<2%) [4]
 Vasculitis [3]
 Wrinkling (sic) [1]
 Xerosis (<2%)

Hair
 Hair – alopecia (<2%)

Nails
 Nails – changes (sic) (<2%)

Cardiovascular
 Flushing (<2%)
 Myocardial infarction [3]
 Myocardial ischemia [1]

Other
 Aphthous stomatitis (<2%)
 Death [3]
 Dizziness (2%) [1]
 Headache

Hyperesthesia (<2%)
Myalgia (<2%) [1]
Oral ulceration (<2%)
Paresthesias (<2%)

Pseudoporphyria [1]
Tendinitis (<2%)
Tinnitus [1]
Xerostomia (<2%)

ROPINIROLE

Trade name: Requip (GSK)
Indications: Parkinsonism
Category: Antiparkinsonian; Dopamine agonist
Half-life: ~6 hours

Reactions

Skin
  Balanitis (<1%)
  Basal cell carcinoma (>1%)
  Cellulitis (<1%)
  Dermatitis (<1%)
  Diaphoresis (6%)
  Eczema (<1%)
  Edema (<1%)
  Exanthems (<1%)
  Fungal dermatitis (<1%)
  Furunculosis (<1%)
  Herpes simplex (<1%)
  Herpes zoster (<1%)
  Hyperkeratosis (<1%)
  Hypertrophy (<1%)
  Peripheral edema (<1%)
  Photosensitivity (<1%)
  Pigmentation (<1%)
  Pruritus (<1%)
  Psoriasis (<1%)
  Purpura (<1%)
  Rash (sic) (>1%)
  Ulcerations (<1%)
  Urticaria (<1%)
  Viral infections

Hair
  Hair – alopecia (<1%)

Cardiovascular
  Flushing (3%)

Other
  Dizziness [1]
  Dyskinesia [1]
  Gingivitis (>1%)
  Glossitis (<1%)
  Gynecomastia (<1%)
  Headache [1]
  Hyperesthesia (4%)
  Mastitis (<1%)
  Paresthesias (5%)
  Peyronie's disease (<1%)
  Sialorrhea (>1%)
  Stomatitis (<1%)
  Thrombophlebitis (<1%)
  Tongue edema (<1%)
  Tremor (6%)
  Ulcerative stomatitis (<1%)
  Vulvovaginal candidiasis (<1%)
  Xerostomia (5%)

RUE

Scientific names: *Ruta chalepensis; Ruta corsica; Ruta graveolens; Ruta montana*
Family: Rutaceae
Trade and other common names: Country man's treacle; Herb of grace; Herbygrass; ruda
Category: Antispasmodic; Emmenagogue
Purported indications and other uses: Hysteria, coughs, croup, colic, flatulence, mild stomachic, insomnia, abdominal cramps, nervous headache, giddiness, hysteria, palpitation, abortifacient, cysticide, vermifuge, insecticide. **Topical:** irritant, rubefacient for eczemas, psoriasis and rheumatic pain, sciatica, headache, chronic bronchitis. Flavoring in alcoholic beverages, salads, meats and cheeses
Half-life: N/A

Reactions

Skin
  Bullous dermatitis [2]
  Clammy skin
  Dermatitis
  Edema
  Erythema [2]

  Photosensitivity [8]
  Vesiculation [2]

Other
  Death
  Seizures

SALSALATE

Synonyms: disalicylic acid; salicylic acid
Trade names: Mono-Gesic (Schwarz); Salflex
Other common trade names: *Argesic-SA; Artha-G; Atisuril; Disalgesic; Marthritic; Nobegyl; Salgesic; Salina; Umbradol*
Indications: Arthritis
Category: Nonsteroidal anti-inflammatory (NSAID) analgesic; Salicylate
Half-life: 7–8 hours
Clinically important, potentially hazardous interactions with: methotrexate

---

Reactions

Skin
  Angioedema
  Dermatitis
  Exanthems
  Lichenoid eruption [1]
  Pruritus
  Purpura
  Rash (sic) (1–10%)

  Urticaria [1]

Nails
  Nails – onychoschizia [1]

Other
  Anaphylactoid reactions (1–10%)
  Tinnitus

SARSAPARILLA

Scientific names: *Smilax aristolochiaefolia; Smilax febrifuga; Smilax glabra; Smilax japicanga; Smilax officinalis; Smilax ornata; Smilax regelii; Smilax rotundifolia*
Family: Smilacaceae
Trade and other common names: Greenbriar; Horsebrier; jupicanga; khao yen; Round-leaf; Salsaparrilha; saparna; smilace; smilax; zarzaparilla
Category: Anti-inflammatory; Antioxidant; Immunomodulator
Purported indications and other uses: blood purifier, general tonic, gout, syphilis, gonorrhea, rheumatism, wounds, arthritis, fever, cough, scrofula, hypertension, digestive disorders, psoriasis, skin diseases, cancer
Half-life: N/A
Clinically important, potentially hazardous interactions with: digoxin

Note: Sarsaparilla vine should not be confused with sasparilla and sassafras (the root and bark of which were once used to flavor root beer). Sarsaparilla is only used in root beer and other beverages for its foaming properties

Reactions

None

SAW PALMETTO

Scientific names: *Sabal serrulata; Serenoa repens; Serenoa serrulata*
Family: Arecaceae; Palmae
Trade and other common names: American Dwarf Palm Tree; Cabbage Palm; Ju-Zhong; Palmier Nain; Sabal Fructus
Category: Anti-inflammatory; Antiseptic
Purported indications and other uses: Benign prostatic hyperplasia, diuretic, sedative, prostate cancer (with other herbs), aphrodisiac, hair growth, colds, coughs, sore throat, asthma, chronic bronchitis, migraine
Half-life: N/A
Clinically important, potentially hazardous interactions with: oral contraceptives, warfarin

Reactions

Skin
  Adverse effects (sic) [3]

Hemorrhage [1]
Sensitization [1]

SCOPOLAMINE

Trade names: Isopto Hyoscine Ophthalmic; Scopase; Transderm-Scop Patch (Novartis)
Other common trade names: *Scopace; Scopoderm-TTS; Transdermal-V*
Indications: Nausea and vomiting, excess salivation
Category: Anticholinergic; Antispasmodic
Half-life: 8 hours
Clinically important, potentially hazardous interactions with: anticholinergics, arbutamine

Reactions

Skin
  Allergic reactions (sic) [1]
  Dermatitis (transdermal patch and
    ophthalmic) [7]
  Edema (<1%) (ophthalmic)
  Erythema
  Erythema multiforme [2]
  Exanthems [1]
  Fixed eruption [1]
  Hypohidrosis (>10%)
  Photosensitivity (1–10%)
  Rash (sic) (<1%)

  Urticaria
  Xerosis (>10%)

Cardiovascular
  Flushing

Other
  Anaphylactoid reactions [2]
  Death
  Dizziness [1]
  Headache
  Injection-site irritation (>10%)
  Oral lesions (>5%) [1]
  Xerostomia (>60%) [3]

Note: Systemic adverse effects have been reported following ophthalmic administration

SELEGILINE

Synonyms: deprenyl; L-deprenyl
Trade name: Eldepryl (Somerset)
Other common trade names: *Apo-Selegiline; Carbex; Eldeprine; Jumex; Movergan; Novo-Selegiline; Plurimen*
Indications: Parkinsonism
Category: Antiparkinsonian; Monoamine oxidase (MAO) inhibitor
Half-life: 9 minutes
Clinically important, potentially hazardous interactions with: carbidopa, carbidopa, citalopram, doxepin, ephedra, ephedrine, escitalopram, fluoxetine, fluvoxamine, levodopa, meperidine, nefazodone, oral contraceptives, paroxetine, sertraline, venlafaxine

Reactions

Skin
  Diaphoresis
  Peripheral edema
  Photosensitivity
  Rash (sic)

Hair
  Hair – alopecia
  Hair – hypertrichosis (facial)

Other
Application-site reactions (sic) [1]
Bruxism (1–10%)
Death [1]
Dysgeusia
Headache
Oral ulceration [1]

Paresthesias
Serotonin syndrome [1]
Stomatitis [1]
Tinnitus
Tremor
Xerostomia (>10%) [1]

SELENIUM

Trade names: Bio-Active Selenium (Solaray); Exsel Shampoo; Head & Shoulders Intensive Treatment Dandruff Shampoo (Procter & Gamble); SelenoMax (Source Naturals); Selsun Blue (Chattem); Selsun Shampoo (Chattem); Vpak51
Other common trade names: *Selenate; Selenite; selenium dioxide; selenium sulfide; selenocysteine; selenomethionine*
Indications: Anticancer (stomach, colorectal, lung, prostate), arthritis, asthma, heart disease, HIV inhibitor. Treatment of dandruff, fungal infections (tinea versicolor), and seborrhea
Category: Essential micronutrient
Half-life: 12–41 hours; Selenomethionine: 252 days, Selinite: 102 days
Clinically important, potentially hazardous interactions with: cholesterol-lowering drugs, cholesterol-lowering drugs, cisplatin, clozapine, dimercaprol, niacin, oral corticosteroids, oral corticosteroids, simvastatin

---

Reactions

Skin
Adverse effects (sic) [2]
Allergic reactions (sic)
Carcinoma [5]
Dermatitis [1]
Diaphoresis
Erythema chronicum persistans [1]
Infections
Lupus erythematosus (from deficiency)
Melanoma [1]
Photosensitivity
Pruritus
Rash (sic)
Scleroderma (deficiency)

Hair
Hair – alopecia [2]
Hair – brittle [1]

Hair – changes (sic) [2]
Hair – pigmentation

Nails
Nails – brittle [4]
Nails – loss [1]
Nails – paronychia
Nails – white streaking

Cardiovascular
Flushing

Other
Amyotrophic lateral sclerosis [4]
Arthralgia (from deficiency)
Death (overdose)
Dysgeusia (metallic taste)
Myalgia
Paresthesias

Sialorrhea	Tremor
Tooth disorder (sic)	

Note: Selenium is an essential component of glutathione peroxidase. Inadequate concentrations of dietry selenium account, in part, for Keshan disease (a fatal cardiomyopathy)

SIBERIAN GINSENG

Scientific names: *Acanthopanax senticosus; Eleutherococcus senticosus*
Family: Araliaceae
Trade and other common names: Ciwulja; Devil's root; Eleuthero; Ezoukogi; Medexport; Shigoka; Taiga Wurzel; Touch-me-not
Category: Adaptogen; Antidementia; Emmenagogue; Immunoregulator
Purported indications and other uses: Alzheimer's disease, anaphylaxis, arthritis, colds, depression, fatigue, flu, impotence, infertility, menopause, multiple sclerosis, osteoporosis, perimenopause, PMS, stress
Half-life: N/A
Clinically important, potentially hazardous interactions with: antihypertensives, digoxin

---
Reactions

Other	Mastodynia
Headache	

Note: Eleutherococcus may prevent biotransformation of some drugs to less toxic compounds

SODIUM OXYBATE

Synonyms: Gamma Hydroxybutyrate; GHB
Trade name: Xyrem (Orphan Medical)
Indications: Cataplexy (in patients with narcolepsy)
Category: Anesthetic; Anticataplectic; CNS depressant; Dietary supplement
Half-life: 0.3–1 hour
Clinically important, potentially hazardous interactions with: alcohol, hypnotics, sedatives

---
Reactions

Skin	Depression
Diaphoresis [3]	Pain
Flu-like syndrome	Porphyria
Infections	Rhabdomyolysis
Upper respiratory infection	Seizures [7]
Other	Sialorrhea
Back pain	Sinusitis
Death [9]	Tremor [4]

Note: Sodium Oxybate is a class of drugs that are also known as: 'Designer' drugs; Party drugs; Club drugs; Recreational drugs; 'Rave' drugs; Fantasy drugs; Date rape drugs; abuse drugs

SOLIFENACIN

Trade name: Vesicare (GSK)
Indications: Overactive bladder
Category: Muscarinic antagonist
Half-life: 45–68 hours
Clinically important, potentially hazardous interactions with: atazanavir, carbamazepine, clarithromycin, indinavir, itraconazole, ketoconazole, nefazodone, nelfinavir, phenobarbital, phenytoin, rifabutin, rifampin, rifapentine, ritonavir, saquinavir, st john's wort, telithromycin, troleandomycin, voriconazole

Reactions

Skin
Pharyngitis (0.3–1.1%)

Eyes
Blurred vision (4–5%)
Xerophthalmia (0.3–1.6%)

Cardiovascular
Hypertension (0.5–1.4%)

Other
Abdominal pain (1.2–1.9%)
Cough (0.2–1.1%)
Depression (0.8–1.2%)
Dizziness (1.9%)
Fatigue (1–2.1%)
Urinary tract infection (3.5%)
Xerostomia (11–27%) [3]

ST JOHN'S WORT

Scientific name: *Hypericum perforatum*
Family: Hypericaceae
Trade and other common names: Amber; Demon Chaser; Fuga Daemonum; Goatweed; Hardhay; Hypereikon; Hypericum; Johns Wort; Klamath Weed; Rosin Rose; Tipton Weed
Category: Anti-anxiety
Purported indications and other uses: Depression, dysthymic disorder, fatigue, insomnia, loss of appetite, anxiety, obsessive-compulsive disorders, mood disturbances, migraine headaches, neuralgia, fibrositis, sciatica, palpitations, exhaustion, headache, muscle pain, vitiligo, diuretic, bruises, abrasions, first degree burns, hemorrhoids
Half-life: N/A
Clinically important, potentially hazardous interactions with: alprazolam, amitriptyline, amprenavir, atazanavir, bosentan, buspirone, carbamazepine, citalopram, cyclosporine, digoxin, eplerenone, escitalopram, etoposide, fexofenadine, fluoxetine, fluvoxamine, fosamprenavir, ginkgo biloba, imatinib, indinavir, irinotecan, loperamide, methadone, midazolam, naratriptan, nefazodone, nelfinavir, nevirapine, oral contraceptives, paroxetine, phenobarbitone, phenprocoumon, phenytoin, quinolones ritonavir, ritonavir, rizatriptan, saquinavir, sertraline, simvastatin, sirolimus, solifenacin, SSRIs, sumatriptan, tacrolimus, tetracyclines, theophylline, tricyclic antidepressants, warfarin, zolmitriptan

Reactions

Skin
Adverse effects (sic) [2]
Allergic reactions (sic) [1]
Erythroderma [1]
Irritation
Photosensitivity [6]
Pruritus [1]

Hair
Hair – alopecia [1]

Other
Bleeding [1]
Hypersensitivity
Paresthesias [1]
Serotonin syndrome [4]
Side effects (sic) [1]
Xerostomia [1]

Note: St. John's wort is a natural source of flavoring in Europe. Although not indigenous to Australia, and long considered a weed, St. John's wort is now grown there as a cash crop and produces 20% of the world's supply

SUCCINYLCHOLINE

Synonym: suxamethonium
Trade name: Anectine (Sabex)
Indications: Skeletal muscle relaxation during general anesthesia
Category: Cholinergic; Skeletal muscle relaxant
Half-life: N/A
Clinically important, potentially hazardous interactions with: amikacin, aminoglycosides, galantamine, gentamicin, kanamycin, neomycin, paromomycin, physostigmine, pipecuronium, streptomycin, tobramycin, vancomycin, vecuronium

Reactions

Skin
  Dermatitis [1]
  Erythema (<1%) [1]
  Exanthems
  Pruritus (<1%)
  Rash (sic) (<1%)
  Urticaria

Cardiovascular
  Bradycardia [1]

Flushing
Tachycardia [1]

Other
  Anaphylactoid reactions [7]
  Hypersensitivity [1]
  Myalgia (<1%) [5]
  Rhabdomyolysis [23]
  Sialorrhea (1–10%)

SUFENTANIL

Trade name: Sufenta (Akorn)
Indications: Epidural and general anesthesia
Category: Narcotic analgesic
Half-life: 152 minutes
Clinically important, potentially hazardous interactions with: cimetidine

Reactions

Skin
  Chills
  Clammy skin (<1%)
  Erythema
  Pruritus [1]

Rash (sic) (<1%)
Urticaria (<1%)

Other
  Dysesthesia (<1%)

SULFASALAZINE

Synonym: salicylazosulfapyridine
Trade name: Azulfidine (Pfizer)
Other common trade names: *Colo-Pleon; Salazopyrin; Salisulf; Saridine; SAS-500; Sulfazine; Ukol*
Indications: Inflammatory bowel disease, ulcerative colitis, rheumatoid arthritis
Category: Sulfonamide
Half-life: 5–10 hours
Clinically important, potentially hazardous interactions with: cholestyramine, methotrexate

---

Reactions

Skin
Acute generalized exanthematous
  pustulosis (AGEP) [4]
Adverse effects (sic) [1]
Angioedema [2]
Bullous eruption
Bullous pemphigoid [1]
Cheilitis [1]
Dermatitis [2]
Diaphoresis [1]
Eczema [1]
Erythema multiforme [8]
Erythema nodosum [2]
Erythroderma [1]
Exanthems (2–23%) [23]
Exfoliative dermatitis [5]
Fixed eruption [7]
Lichen planus [2]
Lupus erythematosus [33]
Necrosis [1]
Photosensitivity (10%) [4]
Pigmentation [3]
Pruritus (10%) [7]
Pruritus ani et vulvae [1]
Psoriasis [1]
Purpura [1]
Pustules [2]
Rash (sic) (>10%) [12]
Raynaud's phenomenon [2]
Side effects (sic) (5%) [1]
Stevens–Johnson syndrome (<1%) [3]
Toxic epidermal necrolysis (1–10%) [11]
Urticaria (1–5%) [11]

Vaginitis [1]
Vasculitis [3]
Xerosis [1]

Hair
Hair – alopecia [6]

Eyes
Periorbital edema

Hematopoietic
Lymphoplasmacytosis [1]

Cardiovascular
Cardiac tamponade [1]
Flushing [2]

Other
Anaphylactoid reactions [3]
Aphthous stomatitis [1]
Death [2]
DRESS syndrome [3]
Dysgeusia [1]
Glossitis
Headache
Hypersensitivity (1–5%) [9]
Hypogeusia
Lymphoproliferative disease [1]
Mononucleosis [1]
Mucocutaneous reactions (6%) [2]
Myalgia [1]
Oral mucosal eruption (<1%) [4]
Oral ulceration [3]
Pseudolymphoma [2]
Serum sickness (<1%) [3]
Stomatitis [1]

Tongue ulceration [1]   Xerostomia [1]

*Note: Sulfasalazine is a sulfonamide and can be absorbed systemically. Sulfonamides can produce severe, possibly fatal, reactions such as toxic epidermal necrolysis and Stevens–Johnson syndrome

SULFINPYRAZONE*

Trade name: Anturane (Novartis)
Other common trade names: *Antazone; Antiran; Anturan; Anturano; Enturen; Falizal; Novopyrazone*
Indications: Gouty arthritis
Category: Antigout; Antihyperuricemic sulfonamide
Half-life: 2–7 hours
Clinically important, potentially hazardous interactions with: anisindione, anticoagulants, dicumarol, warfarin

Reactions

Skin   Purpura
  Dermatitis (1–10%)   Rash (sic) (1–10%)
  Edema
  Exanthems (<3%)   Cardiovascular
                                                      Flushing (<1%)

*Note: Sulfinpyrazone is a sulfonamide and can be absorbed systemically. Sulfonamides can produce severe, possibly fatal, reactions such as toxic epidermal necrolysis and Stevens–Johnson syndrome

SULINDAC

Trade name: Clinoril
Other common trade names: *Aflodac; Algocetil; APO-Sulin; Arthrocine; Mobilin; Novo-Sundac; Sulene; Sulic; Suloril*
Indications: Arthritis
Category: Nonsteroidal anti-inflammatory (NSAID) analgesic
Half-life: 7.8–16.4 hours
Clinically important, potentially hazardous interactions with: methotrexate, warfarin

Reactions

Skin   Exanthems (1–5%) [10]
  Angioedema (<1%)   Exfoliative dermatitis (<1%)
  Dermatitis [1]   Exfoliative erythroderma [1]
  Diaphoresis   Facial erythema [1]
  Edema   Fixed eruption (<1%) [5]
  Erythema [1]   Jaundice [1]
  Erythema multiforme (<1%) [8]   Lichen planus [1]

Pernio [1]
Photosensitivity (<1%) [2]
Phototoxicity
Pruritus (1–10%) [5]
Purpura (<1%) [2]
Rash (sic) (>10%)
Raynaud's phenomenon [1]
Skin pain (sic) [1]
Stevens–Johnson syndrome (<1%) [5]
Toxic epidermal necrolysis (<1%) [13]
Urticaria (<1%) [4]
Vasculitis (<1%)

Hair
Hair – alopecia (<1%)

Hematopoietic
Ecchymoses (<1%)

Cardiovascular
Hot flashes (<1%)

Other
Ageusia (<1%)

Anaphylactoid reactions (<1%) [4]
Aphthous stomatitis
Death
Dysesthesia [1]
Dysgeusia (<1%)
Glossitis (<1%)
Gynecomastia [1]
Headache
Hypersensitivity (<1%) (potentially fatal)
Oral lichenoid eruption [1]
Oral mucosal eruption (3%) [2]
Oral mucosal erythema [1]
Oral ulceration
Paresthesias (<1%)
Pseudolymphoma [1]
Rectal mucosal ulceration [1]
Serum sickness [1]
Stomatitis (<1%) [2]
Tinnitus
Xerostomia [2]

SUMATRIPTAN

Trade name: Imitrex (GSK)
Other common trade name: *Imigrane*
Indications: Migraine attacks
Category: Antimigraine; Serotonin agonist
Half-life: 2.5 hours
Clinically important, potentially hazardous interactions with: citalopram,
dihydroergotamine, ergot-containing drugs, escitalopram, fluoxetine, fluvoxamine, isocarboxazid,
MAO inhibitors, methysergide, naratriptan, nefazodone, paroxetine, phenelzine, rizatriptan,
sertraline, sibutramine, **st john's wort**, tranylcypromine, venlafaxine, zolmitriptan

Reactions

Skin
Angioedema [1]
Burning (1–10%)
Diaphoresis (1.6%)
Erythema (<1%)
Exanthems
Hyperpyrexia [1]
Photosensitivity (<1%)

Pruritus (<1%)
Rash (sic) (<1%)
Raynaud's phenomenon (<1%)
Sensitivity (sic) [1]
Urticaria [1]

Cardiovascular
Atrial fibrillation [1]

Coronary artery disorders [1]
Flushing (6.6%)
Hot flashes (>10%)
Myocardial ischemia [1]

Other
Anaphylactoid reactions
Dysesthesia (<1%)
Dysgeusia (<1%) [1]

Glossodynia
Headache
Hyperesthesia (<1%)
Injection-site reactions (sic) (10–58%) [1]
Myalgia (1.8%)
Parageusia (<1%)
Paresthesias (13.5%)
Parosmia (<1%)
Xerostomia

TEMAZEPAM

Trade names: Restoril (Mallinckrodt); Temazepam
Other common trade names: *Apo-Temazepam; Cerepax; Euhypnos; Lenal; Levanxene; Normison; Nu-Temazepam; Planum*
Indications: Insomnia, anxiety
Category: Benzodiazepine sedative-hypnotic
Half-life: 8–15 hours
Clinically important, potentially hazardous interactions with: amprenavir, chlorpheniramine, clarithromycin, efavirenz, esomeprazole, imatinib, nelfinavir

---

Reactions

Skin
Adverse effects (sic) [1]
Bullous eruption [1]
Dermatitis (1–10%)
Diaphoresis (>10%)
Exanthems
Fixed eruption [1]
Lichenoid eruption [1]
Pruritus
Purpura
Rash (sic) (>10%)

Urticaria

Other
Anaphylactoid reactions [1]
Dysgeusia
Headache
Paresthesias
Sialopenia (>10%)
Sialorrhea (1–10%)
Tremor (<1%)
Xerostomia (1.7%)

THALIDOMIDE

Trade names: Contergan; Distaval; Kevadon; Thalomid (Celgene)
Indications: Graft-versus-host reactions, recalcitrant aphthous stomatitis
Category: Graft-versus-host disease; immunosuppressant
Half-life: 8.7 hours

Reactions

Skin
Adverse effects (sic) [1]
Bullous eruption (5%) [1]
Burning [1]
Dermatitis [1]
Diaphoresis [1]
Edema [7]
Erythema [1]
Erythema nodosum [2]
Erythroderma [2]
Exanthems [3]
Exfoliative dermatitis [2]
Facial erythema (1–5%) [2]
Infections [1]
Neuropathy [2]
Nodular eruption [1]
Palmar erythema [1]
Peripheral edema [2]
Pruritus [2]
Psoriasis [1]
Purpura [1]
Pustuloderma [1]
Rash (sic) (11–50%) [15]
Shaking [1]
Stevens–Johnson syndrome [1]
Toxic epidermal necrolysis [3]

Toxic pustuloderma [1]
Ulcerations [1]
Urticaria (3%) [1]
Vasculitis [1]
Xerosis [4]

Hair
Hair – alopecia [1]

Nails
Nails – brittle [1]

Other
Death [1]
Dizziness [3]
Dysesthesia [1]
Fatigue [2]
Galactorrhea [1]
Gynecomastia [1]
Headache
Hyperesthesia [1]
Hypersensitivity [1]
Neuropathy [4]
Paresthesias [6]
Tremor [1]
Xerostomia [7]

THIOPENTAL

Trade name: Thiopental (Baxter)
Other common trade names: *Anesthal; Hypnostan; Intraval; Nesdonal; Sodipental; Trapanal*
Indications: Induction of anesthesia
Category: Anticonvulsant; Barbiturate anesthetic; Sedative
Half-life: 3–12 hours
Clinically important, potentially hazardous interactions with: ethanol, ethanolamine

Reactions

Skin
  Angioedema [4]
  Bullous eruption [2]
  Erythema (<1%)
  Erythema multiforme [2]
  Exanthems (3%) [3]
  Exfoliative dermatitis
  Fixed eruption [3]
  Hypomelanosis [1]
  Pruritus (<1%)
  Purpura [2]
  Rash (sic)
  Shivering (27%) [1]
  Stevens–Johnson syndrome [1]

  Toxic epidermal necrolysis [1]
  Urticaria [4]

Other
  Anaphylactoid reactions (<1%) [9]
  Headache
  Injection-site necrosis
  Injection-site pain (>10%)
  Injection-site phlebitis (6%) [1]
  Porphyria [4]
  Rhabdomyolysis [1]
  Thrombophlebitis (<1%)
  Twitching (<1%)

TIAGABINE

Trade name: Gabitril (Cephalon)
Indications: Partial seizures
Category: Anticonvulsant
Half-life: 7–9 hours

Reactions

Skin
  Acne (>1%)
  Allergic reactions (sic) (<1%)
  Carcinoma (<1%)
  Dermatitis (<1%)
  Diaphoresis (<1%)
  Eczema (<1%)
  Edema (<1%)
  Exanthems (<1%)
  Exfoliative dermatitis (<1%)

  Facial edema (<1%)
  Furunculosis (<1%)
  Herpes simplex (<1%)
  Herpes zoster (<1%)
  Neoplasms (benign) (<1%)
  Nodular eruption (<1%)
  Peripheral edema (<1%)
  Petechiae (<1%)
  Photosensitivity (<1%)
  Pigmentation (<1%)

Pruritus (2%)
Psoriasis (<1%)
Rash (sic) (5%)
Stevens–Johnson syndrome
Ulcerations (<1%)
Urticaria (<1%)
Vesiculobullous eruption (<1%)
Xerosis (<1%)

Hair
Hair – alopecia (<1%)
Hair – hirsutism (<1%)

Hematopoietic
Ecchymoses (>1%)

Other
Ageusia (<1%)
Depression [1]
Dysgeusia (<1%)

Foetor ex ore (halitosis) (<1%)
Gingival hypertrophy (<1%)
Gingivitis (<1%)
Glossitis (<1%)
Gynecomastia (<1%)
Mastodynia (<1%)
Myalgia (>1%)
Oral ulceration (2%)
Paresthesias (4%)
Parosmia (<1%)
Sialorrhea (<1%)
Stomatitis (<1%)
Thrombophlebitis (<1%)
Tremor (>1%) [2]
Ulcerative stomatitis (<1%)
Vaginitis (<1%)
Xerostomia (>1%)

TIOTROPIUM

Trade name: Spiriva (Boehringer Ingelheim)
Indications: Bronchospasm (associated with COPD)
Category: Anticholinergic (antimuscarinic)
Half-life: 5–6 days

Reactions

Skin
Allergic reactions (sic) (1–3%)
Angioedema (<1%)
Candidiasis (4%)
Edema (5%)
Flu-like syndrome (>3%)
Herpes zoster (1–3%)
Infections
Pruritus
Rash (sic) (4%)
Urticaria

Eyes
Cataract (1–3%)

Cardiovascular
Chest pain (7%)

Other
Abdominal pain (5%)
Arthralgia (>3%)
Bone or joint pain (1–3%)
Cough (>3%)
Depression (1–3%)
Hypersensitivity
Myalgia (4%)
Paresthesias (1–3%)
Pharyngitis (9%)
Rhinitis (6%)
Sinusitis (11%)
Stomatitis (1–3%)
Upper respiratory infection (41%)
Xerostomia (10–16%) [7]

TIZANIDINE

Trade name: Zanaflex (Acorda)
Other common trade names: *Sirdalud; Ternalax; Ternelin*
Indications: Muscle spasticity, multiple sclerosis
Category: Alpha-2-adrenoceptor blocker
Half-life: 2.5 hours

Reactions

Skin
  Acne (<1%)
  Allergic reactions (sic) (<1%)
  Candidiasis (<1%)
  Cellulitis (<1%)
  Diaphoresis (>1%)
  Edema (<1%)
  Exanthems (<1%)
  Exfoliative dermatitis (<1%)
  Herpes simplex (<1%)
  Herpes zoster (<1%)
  Petechiae (<1%)
  Pruritus (1–10%)
  Purpura (<1%)
  Rash (sic) (1–10%)
  Ulcerations (>1%)

  Urticaria (<1%)
  Xerosis (<1%)

Hair
  Hair – alopecia (<1%)

Hematopoietic
  Ecchymoses (<1%)

Cardiovascular
  QT prolongation [1]

Other
  Paresthesias (>1%)
  Tremor (1–10%)
  Vulvovaginal candidiasis (<1%)
  Xerostomia (49%)

TOCAINIDE

Trade name: Tonocard (AstraZeneca)
Indications: Ventricular arrhythmias
Category: Antiarrhythmic class I B
Half-life: 11–14 hours

Reactions

Skin
  Allergic reactions (sic) [2]
  Clammy skin
  Diaphoresis (<1%)
  Erythema multiforme (<1%)
  Exanthems [1]
  Exfoliative dermatitis (<1%)
  Lupus erythematosus (<1%) [2]
  Pallor (<1%)
  Pruritus (<1%)

  Rash (sic) (0.5–8.4%)
  Stevens–Johnson syndrome (<1%)
  Vasculitis (<1%)

Hair
  Hair – alopecia (<1%)

Cardiovascular
  Bradycardia [1]
  Congestive heart failure [1]

Other
  Dysgeusia (8.4%)
  Gingivitis [1]
  Headache
  Hypersensitivity (<1%)
  Myalgia (<1%)

  Paresthesias (3.5–9%)
  Parosmia (<1%)
  Stomatitis (<1%)
  Tinnitus
  Xerostomia (<1%)

TOLCAPONE

Trade name: Tasmar (Roche)
Indications: Parkinsonism
Category: Antiparkinsonian
Half-life: 2–3 hours

Reactions

Skin
  Allergic reactions (sic) (<1%)
  Burning (2%)
  Cellulitis (<1%)
  Diaphoresis (7%)
  Eczema (<1%)
  Edema (<1%)
  Erythema multiforme (<1%)
  Facial edema (<1%)
  Fungal dermatitis (<1%)
  Furunculosis (<1%)
  Herpes simplex (<1%)
  Herpes zoster (<1%)
  Pigmentation (<1%)
  Pruritus (<1%)
  Rash (sic) (<1%)
  Seborrhea (<1%)
  Urticaria (<1%)

  Vitiligo [1]
Hair
  Hair – alopecia (1%)
Other
  Headache
  Hyperesthesia (<1%)
  Myalgia (<1%)
  Oral ulceration (<1%)
  Paresthesias (3%)
  Parosmia (<1%)
  Sialorrhea (<1%)
  Tongue disorder (<1%)
  Tooth disorder (<1%)
  Tumors (1%)
  Twitching (<1%)
  Vaginitis (<1%)
  Xerostomia (5%)

TOLMETIN

Trade name: Tolectin (Ortho-McNeil)
Other common trade names: *Donison; Midocil; Novo-Tolmetin; Reutol; Safitex*
Indications: Arthritis
Category: Nonsteroidal anti-inflammatory (NSAID) analgesic
Half-life: 1–2 hours
Clinically important, potentially hazardous interactions with: methotrexate

Reactions

Skin
 Angioedema (<1%) [2]
 Bullous eruption
 Diaphoresis
 Edema (3–9%)
 Erythema multiforme (<1%)
 Exanthems (9%) [4]
 Photosensitivity [1]
 Pruritus (1–10%) [3]
 Purpura [1]
 Rash (sic) (>10%)
 Stevens–Johnson syndrome (<1%)
 Toxic epidermal necrolysis (<1%) [3]
 Urticaria (1–5%) [5]

Cardiovascular
 Hot flashes (<1%)

Other
 Anaphylactoid reactions [7]
 Aphthous stomatitis
 Dysgeusia
 Gingival ulceration
 Glossitis (<1%)
 Gynecomastia
 Headache
 Myalgia
 Oral ulceration
 Serum sickness (<1%)
 Stomatitis (<1%)
 Tinnitus
 Xerostomia

TOLTERODINE

Trade name: Detrol (Pfizer)
Indications: Urinary incontinence
Category: Anticholinergic; Muscarinic antagonist (overactive bladder)
Half-life: 2–4 hours

Reactions

Skin
 Erythema (1.9%)
 Flu-like syndrome (4.4%)
 Fungal dermatitis (1.1%)
 Pruritus (1.3%)
 Rash (sic) (1.9%)
 Upper respiratory infection (5.9%)

 Xerosis (1.7%)

Other
 Hallucinations [1]
 Headache
 Paresthesias (1.1%)
 Xerostomia (40%) [13]

TOPIRAMATE

Trade name: Topamax (Ortho-McNeil)
Indications: Partial onset seizures
Category: Anticonvulsant
Half-life: 21 hours

Reactions

Skin
Acne (>1%)
Basal cell carcinoma (<1%)
Dermatitis (<1%)
Diaphoresis (1.8%)
Eczema (<1%)
Edema (1.8%)
Exanthems (<1%) [1]
Facial edema (<1%) [1]
Flu-like syndrome (1–10%)
Folliculitis (<1%)
Hypohidrosis (<1%) [2]
Palmar erythema [1]
Photosensitivity (<1%)
Pigmentation (<1%)
Pruritus (1.8%) [1]
Purpura (<1%)
Rash (sic) (4.4%)
Seborrhea (<1%)
Urticaria (<1%)
Xerosis (<1%)

Hair
Hair – abnormal texture (<1%)
Hair – alopecia (>1%) [1]

Nails
Nails – changes (sic) (<1%)

Eyes
Blurred vision [1]
Glaucoma [4]
Myopia [3]

Periorbital edema [1]
Scleritis [1]

Cardiovascular
Flushing (<1%)
Hot flashes (1–10%)

Other
Ageusia (<1%)
Bromhidrosis (1.8%)
Depression [3]
Dizziness (6%) [2]
Dysgeusia (>1%) [3]
Fatigue [2]
Foetor ex ore (halitosis)
Gingival hypertrophy (<1%)
Gingivitis (1.8%)
Gynecomastia (8.3%)
Hyperesthesia (<1%)
Mastodynia (3–9%)
Myalgia (1.8%)
Oligohydrosis [1]
Paresthesias (15%) [11]
Parosmia (<1%)
Seizures [1]
Sialorrhea [1]
Stomatitis (<1%)
Tongue edema (<1%)
Tremor (>10%)
Vaginitis
Xerostomia (2.7%)

TRAMADOL

Trade names: Ultracet (Ortho-McNeil); Ultram (Ortho-McNeil)
Other common trade names: *Contramal; Tadol; Tradol; Tramal; Tramed; Tramol; Tridol; Zipan*
Indications: Pain
Category: Centrally-acting synthetic analgesic
Half-life: 6–7 hours
Clinically important, potentially hazardous interactions with: citalopram, desflurane, fluoxetine, fluvoxamine, MAO inhibitors, nefazodone, phenelzine, tranylcypromine, venlafaxine

Reactions

Skin
 Allergic reactions (sic) (<1%)
 Angioedema [1]
 Diaphoresis (9%) [1]
 Exanthems [1]
 Pruritus (<10%) [2]
 Rash (sic) (1–5%) [1]
 Shivering [1]
 Toxic dermatitis [1]
 Urticaria (1–18%) [1]

Eyes
 Mydriasis [1]

Other
 Anaphylactoid reactions [1]
 Death [1]
 Dysgeusia (<1%)
 Fever [1]
 Headache
 Paresthesias (<1%)
 Seizures [1]
 Serotonin syndrome [4]
 Stomatitis
 Tremor (5–10%)
 Xerostomia (10%) [2]

TRIHEXYPHENIDYL

Other common trade names: *Acamed; Aparkane; Bentex; Hexinal; Hipokinon; Parkines; Partane; Tridyl; Trihexy; Trihexyphen*
Indications: Parkinsonism
Category: Anticholinergic; Antidyskinetic; Antiparkinsonian
Half-life: 3–4 hours
Clinically important, potentially hazardous interactions with: anticholinergics, arbutamine

Reactions

Skin
 Chills
 Diaphoresis
 Hypohidrosis (>10%)
 Photosensitivity (1–10%)
 Rash (sic) (<1%)
 Spider angiomas [1]
 Urticaria
 Xerosis (>10%)

Cardiovascular
 Flushing

Other
 Glossitis
 Glossodynia
 Paresthesias
 Xerostomia (30–50%)

TRIMETHADIONE

Trade name: Tridione
Other common trade name: *Mino Aleviatin*
Category: Anticonvulsant
Half-life: N/A

Reactions

Skin
  Acne
  Bullous eruption
  Erythema multiforme [4]
  Exanthems [3]
  Exfoliative dermatitis [2]
  Fixed eruption
  Infections (3%) [1]
  Lupus erythematosus [6]
  Petechiae
  Photosensitivity [1]
  Pruritus [1]
  Purpura [1]
  Stevens–Johnson syndrome [1]
  Urticaria [3]
  Vasculitis [2]

Hair
  Hair – alopecia [1]

Other
  Acute intermittent porphyria
  Gingivitis
  Mucositis (4%) [1]
  Paresthesias

TRYPTOPHAN

Scientific name: *L-2-amino-3-(indole-3yl) propionic acid*
Family: None
Trade and other common names: 5-HT; 5-HTP; 5-hydroxytryptophan; 5-OHTrp; L-trypt; L-tryptophan
Category: Sedative; Serotonin modulator
Purported indications and other uses: Insomnia, depression, myofascial pain, premenstrual syndrome, smoking cessation, bruxism
Half-life: N/A
Clinically important, potentially hazardous interactions with: fluoxetine, fluvoxamine, isocarboxazid, phenelzine, sibutramine, tranylcypromine

Reactions

Skin
  Diaphoresis (with phenelzine)
  Scleroderma [4]

Other
  Death [1]
  Eosinophilia–myalgia syndrome [17]
  Fever [1]
  Parkinsonism
  Serotonin syndrome [1]
  Shivering (with phenelzine)

Note: Tryptophan is an essential amino acid. It is a precursor of serotonin and is also converted to nicotinic acid and nicotinamide

TURMERIC

Scientific names: *Curcuma aromatica; Curcuma domestica; Curcuma longa; Curcuma xanthorrhiza*
Family: Zingiberaceae
Trade and other common names: Calebin-A; Chiang Huang; Curcumin; E100; Haridra; Indian Saffron; Jiang Huang; Yellow Root; Yu Jin; Zedoary
Category: Anti-inflammatory
Purported indications and other uses: Arthritis, anticarcinogen, stimulant, carminative, amenorrhea, angina, asthma, colorectal cancer, delirium, diarrhea, dyspepsia, flatulence, hemorrhage, hepatitis, hypercholesterolemia, hypertension, jaundice, mania, menstrual disorders, ophthalmia, tendonitis. Topical: conjuctivitis, skin cancer, smallpox, chickenpox, leg ulcers. Food coloring in cheese, margarine, sweets, snack foods, cosmetics, essential oil in perfumes, culinary spice
Half-life: N/A

Reactions

Skin
  Allergic reactions (sic) (rare)
  Dermatitis [3]

Other
  Headache [1]

Note: Persons with symptoms of gallstones or obstruction of bile passages should avoid turmeric

VALPROIC ACID

Trade names: Depacon (Abbott); Depakene (Abbott)
Indications: Seizures, migraine
Category: Anticonvulsant
Half-life: 6–16 hours
Clinically important, potentially hazardous interactions with: aspirin, cholestyramine, ivermectin

Reactions

Skin
  Acne
  Allergic reactions (sic) (<5%)
  Anticonvulsant hypersensitivity syndrome [3]
  Bullous eruption [1]
  Dermatitis
  Diaphoresis [1]
  Edema [1]
  Erythema multiforme (<1%) [2]
  Exanthems (5%) [1]

  Facial edema (>5%)
  Fixed eruption [1]
  Furunculosis (<5%)
  Lupus erythematosus [5]
  Morphea [1]
  Peripheral edema (<5%)
  Petechiae (<5%) [1]
  Photosensitivity [1]
  Pruritus (>5%) [1]
  Psoriasis
  Purpura [2]

Rash (sic) (>5%) [2]
Scleroderma [1]
Seborrhea
Stevens–Johnson syndrome [2]
Toxic epidermal necrolysis [2]
Urticaria
Vasculitis [2]

Hair
Hair – alopecia (7%) [13]
Hair – curly [3]
Hair – depigmentation [1]

Hematopoietic
Ecchymoses (<5%) [4]

Other
Acute intermittent porphyria [2]
Aplasia cutis congenita
Death [2]
Dysgeusia (<5%)
Galactorrhea [1]

Gingival hypertrophy [3]
Glossitis (<5%)
Gynecomastia [1]
Headache
Hyperesthesia
Hypersensitivity [3]
Myalgia (<5%)
Paresthesias (<5%)
Parkinsonism [2]
Porphyria [2]
Pseudolymphoma [1]
Rhabdomyolysis [1]
Seizures [1]
Sialorrhea
Stomatitis (<5%)
Tinnitus [1]
Tremor [3]
Vaginitis (<5%)
Xerostomia (<5%) [1]

VECURONIUM

Trade name: Norcuron
Other common trade name: *Vecuron*
Indications: Adjunct to general anesthesia
Category: Anesthetic; Non-depolarizing neuromuscular blocker; Skeletal muscle relaxant
Half-life: 65–75 minutes
Clinically important, potentially hazardous interactions with: aminoglycosides, gentamicin, halothane, inhalational anesthetics, kanamycin, magnesium salts, neomycin, quinidine, streptomycin, succinylcholine, tobramycin

Reactions

Other
  Anaphylactoid reactions

Injection-site pain [1]

VERAPAMIL

Trade names: Calan (Pfizer); Covera-HS (Pfizer); Isoptin (Abbott); Tarka (Abbott); Verelan (Schwarz)
Other common trade names: *APO-Verap; Arpamyl LP; Azupamil; Berkatens; Chronovera; Cordilox; Geangin; Isoptine; Nu-Verap; Veraken*
Indications: Angina, hypertension
Category: Antianginal; Antihypertensive; Calcium channel blocker
Half-life: 2–8 hours
Clinically important, potentially hazardous interactions with: acebutolol, amiodarone, aspirin, atenolol, atorvastatin, betaxolol, carbamazepine, carteolol, clonidine, dantrolene, digoxin, dofetilide, epirubicin, eplerenone, erythromycin, esmolol, eucalyptus, lovastatin, metoprolol, mistletoe, nadolol, penbutolol, pindolol, propranolol, quinidine, sibutramine, simvastatin, telithromycin, timolol

Tarka is trandolapril and verapamil

Reactions

Skin
  Acne [1]
  Acute febrile neutrophilic dermatosis (Sweet's syndrome) [1]
  Angioedema [3]
  Dermatitis
  Diaphoresis (<1%) [2]
  Edema (1.9%)
  Erythema multiforme (<1%) [4]
  Erythema nodosum [1]
  Exanthems [7]

  Exfoliative dermatitis [2]
  Hyperkeratosis (palms) (<1%) [2]
  Lichenoid eruption
  Lupus erythematosus [2]
  Peripheral edema (1–10%) [1]
  Photosensitivity [4]
  Prurigo [1]
  Pruritus [6]
  Purpura (<1%) [1]
  Rash (sic) (1.2%) [2]
  Side effects (sic) [2]

Stevens–Johnson syndrome (<1%) [4]
Urticaria (<1%) [5]
Vasculitis (<1%) [2]

Hair
Hair – alopecia (<1%) [6]
Hair – hypertrichosis [1]
Hair – pigmentation [1]

Nails
Nails – dystrophy [1]

Hematopoietic
Ecchymoses (<1%) [1]

Cardiovascular
Atrial fibrillation [2]
Bradycardia [5]
Cardiomegaly [1]
Congestive heart failure [1]
Flushing (1–7%) [4]

Hypotension [1]
QT prolongation [1]
Tachycardia [1]

Other
Cough [1]
Dizziness [1]
Dyspnea [1]
Erythromelalgia [1]
Fatigue [1]
Galactorrhea (<1%)
Gingival hypertrophy (19%) [4]
Gynecomastia (<1%) [4]
Headache
Paresthesias (<1%)
Parkinsonism [1]
Rhabdomyolysis [1]
Serum sickness [1]
Xerostomia (<1%)

VIGABATRIN

Trade name: Sabril (Ovation)
Indications: Epilepsy, infantile spasms (West's syndrome)
Category: Anticonvulsant; Antiepileptic
Half-life: 5–8 hours (young adults); 12–13 hours (elderly)
Clinically important, potentially hazardous interactions with: phenytoin

Reactions

Eyes
Dyschromatopsia (blue-yellow)
Eye pain

Other
Abdominal pain (1.4%)
Anxiety
Asthenia (1.1%)
Depression (2.5%) [2]
Dizziness (3.8%)

Fatigue (9.2%)
Gingival hypertrophy [1]
Headache (3.8%) [1]
Joint pains
Paresthesias
Psychosis [3]
Seizures [2]
Sialorrhea
Tremor

WILLOW BARK

Scientific names: *Salix alba; Salix fragilis; Salix purpurea*
Family: Salicaceae
Trade and other common names: Basket Willow; Brittle Willow; Crack Willow; White Willow; Willowbark
Category: Anti-inflammatory; Antinociceptive; Antipyretic
Purported indications and other uses: Colds, infections, headaches, pain, muscle and joint aches, influenza, gouty arthritis, ankylosing spondylitis, rheumatoid arthritis, osteoarthritis
Half-life: N/A
Clinically important, potentially hazardous interactions with: NSAIDs, salicylates

Reactions

Skin	Other
Rash (sic)	Anaphylactoid reactions [1]

YARROW

Scientific name: *Achillea millefolium*
Family: Compositae
Trade and other common names: Angel flower; Bad Man's Plaything; Bloodwort; Carpenter's Weed; Devil's Nettle; Devil's Plaything; Herbe Militaris; Knight's Milfoil; Milfoil; Millefoil; Nose Bleed; Nosebleed; Old Man's Pepper; Sanguinary; Soldier's Woundwort; Staunchgrass; Staunchweed; Thousand Weed; Thousand-leaf; Yarroway
Category: Anti-inflammatory; Antipyretic; Astringent; Diaphoretic; Diuretic; Haemostatic
Purported indications and other uses: Fevers, common cold, essential hypertension, digestive complaints, loss of appetite, amenorrhoea, dysentery, diarrhoea, cerebral and coronary thromboses, menstrual pain, bleeding piles, toothache, muscle spasms, gastrointestinal disorders.
Topical: slow-healing wounds, skin inflammations, cosmetics
Half-life: N/A
Clinically important, potentially hazardous interactions with: anticoagulants hypotensives, antiepileptics, hypertensives

Reactions

Skin	
Allergic reactions (sic) [1]	Urticaria [1]
Dermatitis [4]	**Eyes**
Photosensitivity [1]	Rhinoconjunctivitis [1]
Rash (sic) [1]	

YOHIMBINE

Scientific name: *Pausinystalia yohimbe*
Family: Rubiaceae
Trade and other common names: Actibane (Consolidated Midland); Aphrodyne (Star); Yocon (Palisades); Yohimex (Kramer); Yomax
Category: Anesthetic; Aphrodisiac (purported)
Purported indications and other uses: Impotence, alpha2-adrenergic blocker, orthostatic hypertension
Half-life: 36 minutes
Clinically important, potentially hazardous interactions with: tricyclic antidepressants

---

Reactions

Skin
  Adverse effects (sic) [1]
  Diaphoresis
  Exfoliative dermatitis [1]
  Lupus erythematosus [1]

Cardiovascular
  Flushing

Other
  Death

ZALEPLON

Trade name: Sonata (Wyeth)
Indications: Insomnia
Category: Nonbenzodiazepine sedative-hypnotic
Half-life: 1 hour

Reactions

Skin
  Acne (<1%)
  Cheilitis (<1%)
  Chills (<1%)
  Dermatitis (<1%)
  Diaphoresis (<1%)
  Eczema (<1%)
  Edema (<1%)
  Exanthems (<1%)
  Facial edema (<1%)
  Peripheral edema (1–10%)
  Photosensitivity (1–10%)
  Pigmentation (<1%)
  Pruritus (<1%)
  Psoriasis (<1%)

  Purpura (<1%)
  Pustules (<1%)
  Rash (sic) (<1%)
  Vesiculobullous eruption (<1%)
  Xerosis (<1%)

Hair
  Hair – alopecia (<1%)

Hematopoietic
  Ecchymoses (<1%)

Other
  Ageusia (<1%)
  Aphthous stomatitis (<1%)
  Gingival hemorrhage (<1%)
  Gingivitis (<1%)

Glossitis (<1%)
Headache
Hyperesthesia (<1%)
Mastodynia (<1%)
Myalgia (5%)
Oral ulceration (<1%)
Paresthesias (3%)
Parosmia (2%)

Sialorrhea (<1%)
Stomatitis (<1%)
Thrombophlebitis (<1%)
Tongue pigmentation (<1%)
Tremor (1–10%)
Vaginitis (<1%)
Xerostomia (1–10%)

ZOLMITRIPTAN

Trade name: Zomig (AstraZeneca)
Indications: Migraine attacks
Category: Antimigraine; Serotonin agonist
Half-life: 3 hours
Clinically important, potentially hazardous interactions with: dihydroergotamine, ergot, isocarboxazid, MAO inhibitors, methysergide, naratriptan, phenelzine, rizatriptan, sibutramine, st john's wort, sumatriptan, tranylcypromine

Reactions

Skin
 Allergic reactions (sic) (<1%)
 Diaphoresis (2%)
 Edema (<1%)
 Facial edema (<1%)
 Photosensitivity (<1%)
 Pruritus (<1%)
 Rash (sic) (<1%)
 Urticaria (<1%)

Hematopoietic
 Ecchymoses (<1%)

Cardiovascular
 Flushing

Hot flashes (>10%)

Other
 Headache
 Hyperesthesia (<1%)
 Myalgia (2%)
 Paresthesias (11%) [1]
 Parosmia (<1%)
 Serotonin syndrome [1]
 Thrombophlebitis (<1%)
 Tongue edema (<1%)
 Twitching (<1%)
 Xerostomia (3%) [1]

ZONISAMIDE*

Trade name: Zonegran (Eisai)
Indications: Epilepsy
Category: Anticonvulsant sulfonamide
Half-life: 63 hours
Clinically important, potentially hazardous interactions with: caffeine

Reactions

Skin

Acne (<1%)
Allergic reactions (sic) (<1%)
Diaphoresis (<1%)
Eczema (<1%)
Edema (<1%)
Exanthems (<1%)
Facial edema (<1%)
Lupus erythematosus (<1%)
Peripheral edema (<1%)
Petechiae (<1%)
Pruritus (<1%)
Purpura (2%)
Pustules (<1%)
Rash (sic) (3%)
Stevens–Johnson syndrome [1]
Toxic epidermal necrolysis
Urticaria (<1%)
Vesiculobullous eruption (<1%)
Xerosis (<1%)

Hair

Hair – alopecia (<1%)
Hair – hirsutism (<1%)

Hematopoietic

Ecchymoses (2%)

Other

Dysgeusia (2%)
Gingival hypertrophy (<1%)
Gingivitis (<1%)
Glossitis (<1%)
Gynecomastia (<1%) [1]
Headache
Hyperesthesia (<1%)
Hyperpyrexia [1]
Hypersensitivity
Myalgia (<1%)
Oligohydrosis [4]
Oral ulceration (<1%)
Paresthesias (4%)
Parosmia (<1%)
Restless legs syndrome [1]
Stomatitis (<1%)
Thrombophlebitis (<1%)
Tremor (<1%) [1]
Ulcerative stomatitis (<1%)
Xerostomia (2%)

*Note: Zonisamide is a sulfonamide and can be absorbed systemically. Sulfonamides can produce severe, possibly fatal, reactions such as toxic epidermal necrolysis and Stevens–Johnson syndrome

DRUGS RESPONSIBLE FOR COMMON NEUROLOGICAL REACTIONS

ABDOMINAL PAIN
Aminosalicylic acid
Anagrelide
Anakinra
Anastrozole
Aprepitant
Argatroban
Aripiprazole
Azithromycin
Balsalazide
Bevacizumab
Bicalutamide
Bivalirudin
Bortezomib (13%)
Bretylium
Bumetanide
Cabergoline
Candesartan
Capecitabine (35%)
Carbamazepine
Carmustine
Caspofungin
Cefaclor
Cefadroxil
Cefdinir
Cefditoren
Cefixime
Cefpodoxime
Cefprozil
Ceftibuten
Ceftriaxone
Cefuroxime
Celecoxib
Cephalexin
Cetirizine
Cetuximab (26%)
Cevimeline
Chlorotrianisene

Chlorthalidone
Cidofovir
Cinoxacin
Ciprofloxacin
Citalopram
Cladribine
Clarithromycin
Clindamycin
Clofarabine (36%)
Clofazimine (>10%)
Clofibrate
Clomiphene
Clomipramine (>10%)
Clonazepam (>10%)
Clonidine
Clopidogrel
Clotrimazole
Cocaine
Colchicine (>10%)
Colestipol
Corticosteroids
Cyclobenzaprine
Cyclophosphamide
Cyclosporine
Cyproheptadine
Daclizumab
Dapsone
Darbepoetin alfa
Demeclocycline
Denileukin
Dextromethorphan
Diazoxide
Diclofenac
Dicloxacillin
Dicumarol
Didanosine
Digoxin
Dihydroergotamine

Dihydrotachysterol
Dimenhydrinate
Dinoprostone
Diphenhydramine
Dipyridamole
Dirithromycin
Disopyramide
Docetaxel
Dofetilide
Doxazosin
Doxercalciferol
Doxorubicin
Doxycycline
Duloxetine
Efavirenz
Eflornithine
Eletriptan
Emtricitabine (14%)
Enalapril
Enflurane
Enfuvirtide
Enoxaparin
Entacapone
Epirubicin
Eplerenone
Eprosartan
Ergocalciferol
Ertapenem
Erythromycin
Escitalopram
Esomeprazole
Estrogens
Etanercept
Ethambutol
Ethchlorvynol
Ethionamide
Ethotoin
Etodolac
Etoposide
Exemestane
Ezetimibe
Famotidine
Felbamate
Fenofibrate

Fenoldopam
Fenoprofen
Finasteride
Flecainide
Fluconazole
Flucytosine
Fludarabine
Fluorides
Fluoxetine
Fluoxymesterone
Fluphenazine
Flurbiprofen
Flutamide
Fluvastatin
Fluvoxamine
Fondaparinux
Fosamprenavir (5–11%)
Fosfomycin
Fosinopril
Fosphenytoin
Frovatriptan
Fulvestrant (12%)
Furazolidone
Gabapentin
Gadodiamide
Galantamine
Ganciclovir (18%)
Ganirelix
Gatifloxacin
Gefitinib
Gemfibrozil
Gemifloxacin
Gemtuzumab (29%)
Glimepiride
Glipizide
Glyburide
Gold
Granisetron
Granulocyte colony-stimulating factor
(GCSF)
Griseofulvin
Guarana
Halothane
Hepatitis B vaccine

Hyaluronic acid
Hydroxychloroquine
Hydroxyurea
Ibritumomab (16%)
Ibuprofen
Idarubicin
Imatinib (23–37%)
Imiglucerase
Imipenem/Cilastatin
Imipramine
Imiquimod
Immune globulin IV
Inamrinone
Indinavir (14%)
Indomethacin
Infliximab (12%)
Influenza vaccines
Interferon alfa-2A
Interferon beta-1A
Interferon beta-1B (19%)
Isoflurane
Isoniazid
Isotretinoin
Itraconazole
Ivermectin
Ketamine
Ketoconazole
Ketoprofen
Lamivudine
Lamotrigine
Lansoprazole
Laronidase
Leflunomide
Letrozole
Levalbuterol
Levetiracetam
Levodopa
Levofloxacin
Lincomycin
Linezolid
Lisinopril
Lomefloxacin
Loracarbef
Losartan

Lovastatin
Mebendazole
Mecamylamine
Meclizine
Meclofenamate
Medroxyprogesterone
Mefenamic acid
Mefloquine
Meloxicam
Memantine
Mephenytoin
Mercaptopurine
Mesalamine (18%)
Mesoridazine
Metaxalone
Methicillin
Methimazole
Methocarbamol
Methohexital
Methotrexate
Methoxyflurane
Methyldopa
Methylphenidate
Methyltestosterone
Methysergide
Metoclopramide
Metronidazole
Mezlocillin
Miconazole
Midodrine
Mifepristone (96%)
Miglitol (12%)
Miglustat (18–50%)
Minocycline
Mirtazapine
Misoprostol (>10%)
Mitoxantrone
Moexipril
Montelukast
Moxifloxacin
Mupirocin
Myrrh
Nabumetone (12%)
Nafcillin

Nalidixic acid
Naltrexone
Naproxen
Naratriptan
Natalizumab
Nateglinide
Nedocromil
Nefazodone
Nelfinavir
Nesiritide
Nevirapine
Niacin
Nicotine
Nitazoxanide
Nitrofurantoin
Nizatidine
Norfloxacin
Nystatin
Octreotide (>30%)
Ofloxacin
Olanzapine
Olmesartan
Olsalazine (>10%)
Omeprazole
Orlistat (26%)
Orphenadrine
Oseltamivir
Oxacillin
Oxaliplatin (31%)
Oxaprozin (12%)
Oxcarbazepine (10–13%)
Oxybutynin
Oxycodone
Oxytetracycline
Palivizumab
Palonosetron
Pantoprazole
Paramethadione
Paroxetine
Peginterferon alfa-2B (15%)
Pegvisomant
Pemetrexed
Pemirolast
Pemoline

Penicillamine
Penicillins
Pentagastrin
Pentamidine
Pentazocine
Pentosan
Pergolide
Perindopril
Perphenazine
Phenazopyridine
Phenytoin
Physostigmine
Pilocarpine
Pioglitazone
Piperacillin
Piroxicam
Potassium iodide
Pravastatin
Praziquantel
Primaquine
Procarbazine (>10%)
Prochlorperazine
Procyclidine
Progestins
Promazine
Promethazine
Propantheline
Propofol
Propoxyphene
Propylthiouracil
Quetiapine
Quinapril
Quinethazone
Quinidine
Quinine
Rabeprazole
Raloxifene
Ramipril
Ranitidine
Rasburicase (20%)
Reserpine
Reteplase
Rifabutin
Rifapentine

Riluzole
Rimantadine
Risedronate (11%)
Risperidone
Ritonavir
Rituximab (14%)
Rivastigmine (13%)
Rizatriptan
Ropinirole
Rosiglitazone
Rosuvastatin
Salsalate
Saquinavir
Secretin
Sibutramine
Simvastatin
Sirolimus
Sparfloxacin
Spironolactone
Stavudine
Streptokinase
Sulfadoxine
Sulfasalazine
Sulindac
Sumatriptan
Tacrine
Tacrolimus
Tamoxifen
Tegaserod
Telithromycin
Tenecteplase
Tenofovir
Terazosin
Terbinafine
Terbutaline
Terconazole
Tetracycline
Theophylline
Thioguanine
Thiopental
Thioridazine
Thiotepa
Tiagabine
Ticarcillin

Ticlopidine
Tinzaparin
Tiopronin
Tiotropium
Tizanidine
Tocainide
Tolmetin
Tolterodine
Topiramate
Topotecan
Torsemide
Trazodone
Trimetrexate
Trimipramine
Urofollitropin
Valdecoxib
Valganciclovir
Valsartan
Vancomycin
Vasopressin
Vigabatrin
Vincristine
Vinorelbine
Voriconazole
Warfarin
Zalcitabine
Zidovudine
Ziprasidone
Zolmitriptan
Zonisamide

APHASIA
Alemtuzumab
Balsalazide
Carmustine (18%)
Cevimeline
Galantamine
Naproxen
Oxcarbazepine
Primaquine
Progestins
Rivastigmine
Sirolimus
Streptokinase

Telithromycin
Temazepam
Zalcitabine

ASTERIXIS
Bumetanide
Carbamazepine
Ceftazidime
Imipramine
Lithium

ASTHENIA
Abarelix (10%)
Acamprosate (5%)
Acetazolamide
Acetohexamide
Acitretin (1–10%)
Adefovir
Albuterol
Aldesleukin (10–23%)
Alemtuzumab (13–34%)
Alfuzosin (3%)
Alglucerase
Amlodipine
Almotriptan
Alosetron
Alprazolam (10–49%)
Alprostadil (<1%)
Altretamine (1%)
Amantadine (1–5%)
Amiloride
Aminocaproic acid
Amiodarone
Amitriptyline
Amlodipine
Amoxapine
Amphotericin B
Ampicillin
Amprenavir
Anagrelide
Anastrozole
Anthrax vaccine
Apomorphine
Apraclonidine

Aprepitant
Aprotinin
Aripiprazole
Arsenic
Ascorbic acid
Asparaginase
Atazanavir
Atenolol
Atomoxetine
Azacitidine
Azithromycin
Aztreonam
Baclofen
Balsalazide
Basiliximab
Benazepril
Bendroflumethiazide
Bepridil
Bethanechol
Bevacizumab
Bexarotene
Bicalutamide
Bimatoprost
Bismuth
Bleomycin
Bortezomib (65%)
Bosentan
Botulinum toxin (a & b)
Bromocriptine
Bumetanide
Bupropion
Buspirone
Cabergoline
Calcitonin
Candesartan
Capecitabine (42%)
Captopril
Carbamazepine (>10%)
Carbinoxamine
Carboplatin
Carmustine (22%)
Carteolol
Carvedilol (11–24%)
Cascara

Cefdinir
Cefditoren
Cefpodoxime
Ceftibuten
Celecoxib
Cephalexin
Cetirizine
Cetuximab (48%)
Cevimeline
Chasteberry
Chlorambucil
Chlordiazepoxide
Chloroquine
Chlorothiazide
Chlorotrianisene
Chlorthalidone
Chlorzoxazone
Cidofovir (43%)
Cinacalcet
Cinoxacin
Ciprofloxacin
Cisplatin
Citalopram
Cladribine (45%)
Clemastine
Clofarabine (36%)
Clofazimine
Clofibrate
Clomiphene
Clomipramine (>10%)
Clonazepam (>10%)
Clonidine
Clopidogrel
Clorazepate
Clozapine
Co-Trimoxazole
Codeine
Colchicine
Colestipol
Collagen
Corticosteroids
Cyanocobalamin
Cyclobenzaprine
Cyproheptadine

Cyclophosphamide
Cycloserine
Cyclosporine
Cytarabine
Dacarbazine
Daclizumab
Dactinomycin
Danazol
Dantrolene
Daptomycin
Darbepoetin alfa
Delavirdine
Demeclocycline
Denileukin (66%)
Desloratadine
Dextroamphetamine
Diazepam
Dicumarol
Dicyclomine
Didanosine
Diethylpropion
Diethylstilbestrol
Digoxin
Dihydroergotamine
Dihydrotachysterol
Diltiazem
Dimenhydrinate
Diphenhydramine
Dipyridamole
Dirithromycin
Disopyramide
Disulfiram
Dobutamine
Docetaxel
Docusate
Dofetilide
Dolasetron
Donepezil
Dornase alfa
Dorzolamide
Doxacurium
Doxazosin (10–17%)
Doxepin
Doxercalciferol (28%)

Doxorubicin
Dronabinol
Duloxetine (10%)
Dutasteride
Edrophonium
Efalizumab
Efavirenz
Eflornithine
Emtricitabine
Enfuvirtide
Enalapril
Enflurane
Enfuvirtide
Enoxaparin
Entacapone
Ephedrine
Epinephrine
Epirubicin
Eplerenone
Epoetin alfa
Eprosartan
Ergocalciferol
Ertapenem
Erythromycin
Escitalopram
Esmolol
Esomeprazole
Estazolam
Estramustine
Estrogens
Etanercept
Ethacrynic acid
Ethambutol
Ethchlorvynol
Ethosuximide
Ethotoin
Etodolac
Etoposide
Eucalyptus
Exemestane (22%)
Ezetimibe
Famciclovir
Famotidine
Felbamate

Felodipine
Fenofibrate
Fentanyl
Fexofenadine
Flecainide
Fluconazole
Flucytosine
Fludarabine
Flumazenil
Fluorouracil
Fluoxetine
Fluoxymesterone
Fluvoxamine
Fluphenazine
Flurazepam
Flurbiprofen
Flutamide
Fluvastatin
Fluvoxamine
Folic acid
Fondaparinux
Fosamprenavir (10–18%)
Foscarnet
Fosfomycin
Fosinopril
Fosphenytoin
Frovatriptan
Fulvestrant
Furosemide
Gabapentin
Gadodiamide
Galantamine
Ganciclovir
Gatifloxacin
Gefitinib
Gemcitabine (18%)
Gemfibrozil
Gemifloxacin
Gemtuzumab (45%)
Glatiramer (41%)
Glimepiride
Glipizide
Glucagon
Glucosamine

Glyburide
Glycopyrrolate
Gold
Goserelin
Granisetron
Granulocyte colony-stimulating factor (GCSF) (31%)
Griseofulvin
Guanabenz
Guanadrel
Guanfacine
Haloperidol
Halothane
Hepatitis B vaccine
Hydralazine
Hydrochlorothiazide
Hydrocodone
Hydroflumethiazide
Hydroxychloroquine
Hydroxyurea
Hydroxyzine
Hyoscyamine
Ibandronate
Ibuprofen
Ifosfamide
Imatinib (5–41%)
Ibritumomab
Imiglucerase
Imipenem/Cilastatin
Imipramine
Imiquimod
Immune globulin IV
Indapamide
Indinavir
Indomethacin
Infliximab
Influenza vaccines
Insulin
Interferon beta-1b
Interferon alfa-2A (90%)
Interferon beta-1A (40%)
Interferon beta-1B (61%)
Irbesartan
Irinotecan (76%)

Isoetharine
Isoflurane
Isoniazid
Isosorbide dinitrate
Isosorbide mononitrate
Isotretinoin
Isradipine
Itraconazole
Ivermectin
Ketamine
Ketoconazole
Ketoprofen
Labetalol
Lamivudine (>10%)
Lamotrigine
Laronidase
Leflunomide
Letrozole (6–13%)
Levalbuterol
Levamisole
Levetiracetam (15%)
Levodopa
Levofloxacin
Levothyroxine
Liothyronine
Lisinopril
Lithium
Lomefloxacin
Lomustine
Loperamide
Lorazepam
Losartan
Lovastatin
Maprotiline
Mazindol
Mebendazole
Mecamylamine
Mechlorethamine
Meclizine
Meclofenamate
Medroxyprogesterone
Mefenamic acid
Mefloquine
Meloxicam

Memantine
Mepenzolate
Meperidine
Mephenytoin
Mercaptopurine
Mesalamine
Mesoridazine
Metaxalone
Metformin
Methadone
Methamphetamine
Methantheline
Methazolamide
Methocarbamol
Methohexital
Methotrexate
Methoxsalen
Methoxyflurane
Methsuximide
Methyclothiazide
Methyldopa
Methyltestosterone
Metipranolol
Metoclopramide
Metolazone
Metoprolol
Metronidazole
Mexiletine
Midodrine
Mifepristone
Miglustat
Minocycline
Mirtazapine
Misoprostol
Mitomycin
Mitotane (12%)
Modafinil
Moexipril
Molindone
Montelukast
Moricizine
Morphine (>10%)
Moxifloxacin
Mycophenolate (35–43%)

Myrrh
Nabumetone
Nadolol
Nafarelin
Nalbuphine (>10%)
Nalidixic acid
Naproxen
Naratriptan
Natalizumab
Nateglinide
Nedocromil
Nefazodone (>10%)
Nelfinavir
Nesiritide
Nevirapine
Niacin
Nicardipine
Nicotine
Nifedipine (10–12%)
Nitazoxanide
Nitisinone
Nitrofurantoin
Nitroglycerin
Nizatidine
Norfloxacin
Nortriptyline
Octreotide
Ofloxacin
Olanzapine (>10%)
Olmesartan
Omalizumab
Olopatadine
Olsalazine
Omeprazole
Ondansetron (<13%)
Orlistat
Orphenadrine
Oseltamivir
Oxaliplatin (61%)
Oxaprozin
Oxazepam
Oxcarbazepine (12–15%)
Oxycodone (10%)
Paclitaxel

Palivizumab
Palonosetron
Pamidronate (12%)
Pancuronium
Pantoprazole
Paramethadione
Paroxetine (>10%)
Pemetrexed
Papaverine
Peginterferon alfa-2B
Pegvisomant
Pemetrexed (80–87%)
Pemoline
Penbutolol
Penicillamine
Pentagastrin
Pentazocine
Pentosan
Pentostatin
Perflutren
Pergolide
Perindopril
Perphenazine
Phenazopyridine
Phendimetrazine
Phenelzine
Phenoxybenzamine
Phentermine
Phentolamine
Phenytoin
Physostigmine
Pilocarpine
Pimozide
Pindolol
Pioglitazone
Piroxicam
Plicamycin
Polythiazide
Potassium iodide
Pramipexole (>10%)
Pravastatin
Prazepam
Praziquantel
Prazosin

Primidone
Probenecid
Procainamide
Procarbazine (>10%)
Prochlorperazine
Procyclidine
Progestins
Promazine
Promethazine
Propantheline
Propofol
Propoxyphene
Propranolol
Protamine sulfate
Protriptyline
Pseudoephedrine
Pyrazinamide
Pyrimethamine
Quetiapine
Quinapril
Quinethazone
Quinidine
Rabeprazole
Raloxifene
Ramipril
Ranitidine
Rasburicase
Repaglinide
Reserpine
Reteplase
Ribavirin
Rifabutin
Rifampin
Rifapentine
Rifaximin
Riluzole
Rimantadine
Risedronate
Risperidone
Ritodrine
Ritonavir (>10%)
Rituximab (26%)
Rivastigmine
Rizatriptan

Ropinirole (11%)
Rosiglitazone
Rosuvastatin
Salsalate
Saquinavir
Sargramostin
Secretin
Sertraline
Simvastatin
Sirolimus
Sodium oxybate
Solifenacin
Somatropin
Sotalol
Spironolactone
St John's wort
Stavudine
Streptozocin
Sulfadiazine
Sulfadoxine
Sulfamethoxazole
Sulfasalazine
Sulfites
Tadalafil
Tacrolimus
Tamoxifen
Tartrazine
Tegaserod
Telithromycin
Temazepam
Temozolomide
Tenecteplase
Tenofovir
Terazosin
Terbinafine
Terbutaline
Teriparatide
Thalidomide
Thiabendazole
Thioguanine
Thiopental
Thiotepa
Tiagabine
Ticlopidine

Tinidazole
Tizanidine
Tinzaparin
Tiopronin
Tocainide
Tolazamide
Tolbutamide
Topiramate
Topotecan
Toremifene
Torsemide
Tramadol
Trandolapril
Tranylcypromine
Trazodone
Trastuzumab
Travoprost
Treprostinil
Triamterene
Triazolam
Trichlormethiazide
Trientine
Trimethobenzamide
Trimetrexate
Trimipramine
Tripelennamine
Triptorelin
Unoprostone
Urofollitropin
Ursodiol
Valdecoxib
Valganciclovir
Valsartan
Vancomycin
Vasopressin
Venlafaxine
Verapamil
Vigabatrin
Vinblastine
Vincristine
Vinorelbine
Voriconazole
Warfarin
Zafirlukast

Zalcitabine
Zidovudine
Zileuton
Ziprasidone
Zoledronic acid
Zolmitriptan
Zonisamide

ATAXIA

Acetazolamide
Acyclovir (<1%)
Agalsidase
Alprazolam (10–40%)
Altretamine
Amantadine (1–5%)
Amiodarone
Amitriptyline
Amlodipine
Amoxapine
Aripiprazole
Baclofen
Balsalazide
Bevacizumab
Bexarotene
Bortezomib
Bromocriptine
Bupropion
Buspirone
Capecitabine
Captopril
Carbamazepine (>10%)
Carisoprodol
Carmustine
Celecoxib
Cetirizine
Chloral hydrate
Chlorambucil
Chlordiazepoxide (>10%)
Chlorpromazine
Ciprofloxacin
Citalopram
Clemastine
Clomipramine
Clonidine

Clorazepate
Clozapine
Co-Trimoxazole
Cyanocobalamin
Delavirdine
Denileukin
Desipramine
Diazepam
Dicyclomine
Diethylstilbestrol
Diphenhydramine
Dipyridamole
Doxazosin
Doxepin
Dronabinol
Duloxetine
Epoetin alfa
Eprosartan
Escitalopram
Estazolam
Estramustine
Ethionamide
Ethotoin
Eucalyptus
Felbamate
Flecainide
Flucytosine
Flumazenil
Fluorouracil
Flurazepam
Fluvoxamine
Fosphenytoin (<10%)
Frovatriptan
Gabapentin (12%)
Gadodiamide
Galantamine
Ganciclovir
Gatifloxacin
Gentamicin
Glycopyrrolate
Hydroxychloroquine
Hyoscyamine
Imipramine
Immune globulin IV

Influenza vaccines
Interferon beta-1A
Interferon beta-1B (21%)
Irinotecan
Lamotrigine (22%)
Levetiracetam
Levofloxacin
Lindane
Lisinopril
Lithium
Lomefloxacin
Loxapine
Mefloquine
Memantine
Mepenzolate
Mephenytoin
Meprobamate
Mirtazapine
Mesoridazine
Methantheline
Methazolamide
Metronidazole
Mexiletine (10–20%)
Mirtazapine
Moexipril
Moxifloxacin
Nefazodone
Nisoldipine
Norfloxacin
Nortriptyline
Ofloxacin
Olanzapine
Oxazepam
Oxcarbazepine (5–31%)
Paclitaxel
Pemoline
Perindopril
Perphenazine
Phenelzine
Phenytoin
Prazepam
Primidone
Procarbazine (>10%)
Prochlorperazine

Procyclidine
Promazine
Promethazine
Protriptyline
Quazepam
Quinapril
Quinethazone
Quinidine
Ramipril
Rifampin
Selegiline
Sertraline
Tacrine
Tea tree
Telithromycin
Thioguanine
Thioridazine
Thiothixene
Tiagabine
Tinidazole
Topiramate
Trifluoperazine
Trimethobenzamide
Vigabatrin
Vinblastine
Vincristine
Zalcitabine
Zaleplon
Ziprasidone
Zonisamide

BACK PAIN
Alprostadil (1–10%)
Amiloride
Amlodipine
Amphotericin B
Anagrelide
Anastrozole
Apomorphine
Arbutamine
Argatroban
Aripiprazole
Arsenic
Balsalazide

Basiliximab
Bexarotene
Bicalutamide
Bivalirudin (42%)
Bortezomib (14%)
Botulinum toxin (a & b)
Calcitonin
Candesartan
Capecitabine (10%)
Carmustine
Carvedilol
Cefaclor
Celecoxib
Cetirizine
Cetuximab (10%)
Cevimeline
Cilostazol
Clofarabine (13%)
Clofibrate
Clopidogrel
Cyanocobalamin
Cyclophosphamide
Cytarabine
Daclizumab
Dactinomycin
Dalteparin
Danaparoid
Dapsone
Daptomycin
Darbepoetin alfa
Daunorubicin
Denileukin
Dextroamphetamine
Dicumarol
Dihydroergotamine
Dinoprostone
Dipyridamole
Dofetilide
Doxazosin
Doxorubicin
Duloxetine
Efalizumab
Efavirenz
Enflurane

Enoxaparin
Entacapone
Epirubicin
Estramustine
Estrogens
Etanercept
Ethacrynic acid
Etodolac
Etoposide
Exemestane
Ezetimibe
Fenofibrate
Fenoldopam
Fexofenadine
Finasteride
Floxuridine
Fluorides
Fluorouracil
Fomepizole
Fondaparinux
Fosfomycin
Fosphenytoin
Frovatriptan
Fulvestrant (14%)
Gabapentin
Gadodiamide
Galantamine
Gatifloxacin
Gemcitabine
Gemfibrozil
Gemifloxacin
Gemtuzumab (18%)
Glatiramer (16%)
Gold
Granulocyte colony-stimulating factor (GCSF)
Halothane
Heparin
Hepatitis B vaccine
Hyaluronic acid
Hydrochlorothiazide
Hydroflumethiazide
Ibandronate (13%)
Ibritumomab

Ibuprofen
Ifosfamide
Imatinib (10%)
Imiglucerase
Imiquimod
Immune globulin IV
Indomethacin
Infliximab
Interferon alfa-2A
Interferon beta-1A (25%)
Isoflurane
Itraconazole
Ketamine
Ketoconazole
Lamotrigine
Latanoprost
Leflunomide
Letrozole (18%)
Levamisole
Levetiracetam
Levobupivacaine
Levodopa
Levofloxacin
Lidocaine
Lomefloxacin
Lomustine
Loratadine
Losartan
Mechlorethamine
Medroxyprogesterone
Melphalan
Memantine
Mephenytoin
Mercaptopurine
Mesalamine
Methamphetamine
Methenamine
Methohexital
Methotrexate
Methoxyflurane
Methyclothiazide
Midodrine
Miglustat
Mirtazapine

Mitomycin
Mitoxantrone
Modafinil
Moxifloxacin
Mycophenolate (35–47%)
Nalidixic acid
Naproxen
Natalizumab
Nelfinavir
Nesiritide
Nitisinone
Norfloxacin
Ofloxacin
Olanzapine
Olmesartan
Olsalazine
Omeprazole
Orlistat (14%)
Oxaliplatin (11%)
Oxcarbazepine
Paclitaxel
Palonosetron
Pamidronate
Pantoprazole
Paroxetine
Peginterferon alfa-2B
Pegvisomant
Pemirolast
Pentostatin
Pergolide
Perindopril
Phenindamine
Phenytoin
Piroxicam
Polythiazide
Primaquine
Probenecid
Procarbazine
Progestins
Propantheline
Propofol
Protamine sulfate
Quetiapine
Quinapril

Quinine
Ramipril
Rasburicase
Repaglinide
Rifapentine
Riluzole
Risperidone
Rituximab
Rosiglitazone
Rosuvastatin
Sargramostin
Sibutramine
Sirolimus
Streptokinase
Sulfadoxine
Sulfasalazine
Sulfinpyrazone
Tacrolimus
Tadalafil
Tegaserod
Telmisartan
Temazepam
Tenecteplase
Terazosin
Thiabendazole
Thioguanine
Thiopental
Tinidazole
Tinzaparin
Tirofiban
Tizanidine
Topiramate
Tranylcypromine
Travoprost
Triazolam
Triptorelin
Valganciclovir
Valsartan
Vinblastine
Vinorelbine
Zalcitabine
Zidovudine
Zoledronic acid
Zolmitriptan

BELL'S PALSY
Zalcitabine

BLINDNESS
Sirolimus

BONE PAIN
Anastrozole
Aripiprazole
Arsenic
Bexarotene
Bicalutamide
Bortezomib (14%)
Capecitabine
Clofazimine
Cytarabine
Dihydrotachysterol
Doxercalciferol
Ergocalciferol
Etidronate
Exemestane
Fluorides
Fulvestrant (16%)
Gatifloxacin
Glatiramer
Goserelin
Granulocyte colony-stimulating factor (GCSF)
Ibandronate
Imatinib
Interferon beta-1A (10%)
Irbesartan
Letrozole (22%)
Leuprolide
Levofloxacin
Lomefloxacin
Moxifloxacin
Naratriptan
Norfloxacin
Ofloxacin
Pamidronate
Peginterferon alfa-2B
Pegfilgrastim (26%)
Rifampin

Risedronate
Sirolimus
Topiramate
Toremifene
Vinblastine
Zalcitabine
Zoledronic acid

BREAST PAIN

Anastrozole
Celecoxib
Ciprofloxacin
Diethylstilbestrol
Dipyridamole
Domperidone
Eplerenone

BRUXISM

Bupropion
Citalopram
Cocaine
Escitalopram
Indinavir
Levodopa
MDMA
Methylphenidate
Paroxetine
Quetiapine

CHEST PAIN

Amiloride
Amlodipine
Amphotericin B
Ampicillin
Anagrelide
Anastrozole
Apomorphine
Apraclonidine
Aprotinin
Argatroban
Arsenic
Baclofen
Balsalazide
Basiliximab

Bexarotene
Bicalutamide
Bleomycin
Botulinum toxin (a & b)
Brinzolamide
Bumetanide
Bupropion
Candesartan
Capecitabine (6%)
Captopril
Carbinoxamine
Carmustine
Carteolol
Cefaclor
Cefdinir
Cefpodoxime
Cefuroxime
Celecoxib
Cetirizine
Cevimeline
Chlorotrianisene
Cinacalcet
Ciprofloxacin
Citalopram
Clopidogrel
Clozapine
Cyclosporine
Cytarabine
Daclizumab
Danazol
Dantrolene
Darbepoetin alfa
Delavirdine
Denileukin (24%)
Desmopressin
Diazoxide
Dicumarol
Dicyclomine
Diethylpropion
Diflunisal
Dihydroergotamine
Diltiazem
Dipyridamole
Disopyramide

Dobutamine
Docetaxel
Dofetilide
Donepezil
Dornase alfa
Doxazosin
Doxorubicin
Eletriptan
Enalapril
Enfuvirtide
Enoxaparin
Ephedrine
Epinephrine
Eplerenone
Epoetin alfa
Ertapenem
Esmolol
Estramustine
Estrogens
Etanercept
Ethanolamine
Etodolac
Exemestane
Ezetimibe
Felbamate
Fenofibrate
Fenoldopam
Flecainide
Flucytosine
Fludarabine
Flumazenil
Fluorides
Fluorouracil
Fluphenazine
Flurbiprofen
Flutamide
Fondaparinux
Formoterol
Foscarnet
Fosinopril
Frovatriptan
Gabapentin
Gadodiamide
Galantamine

Gatifloxacin
Gemcitabine
Gemifloxacin
Glatiramer (21%)
Glimepiride
Glipizide
Glyburide
Glycopyrrolate
Goserelin
Granisetron
Granulocyte colony-stimulating factor (GCSF)
Guanadrel
Guanfacine
Heparin
Hydralazine
Ibandronate
Ibritumomab
Ibuprofen
Imiquimod
Immune globulin IV
Inamrinone
Indomethacin
Interferon alfa-2A (4–11%)
Interferon beta-1A
Interferon beta-1B (11%)
Irinotecan
Isocarboxazid
Isotretinoin
Isoxsuprine
Itraconazole
Ketoconazole
Ketoprofen
Labetalol
Lamotrigine
Lansoprazole
Laronidase
Latanoprost
Leflunomide
Letrozole
Leuprolide
Levalbuterol
Levofloxacin
Lisinopril

Lomefloxacin
Loratadine
Losartan
Lovastatin
Mazindol
Meclofenamate
Medroxyprogesterone
Mefenamic acid
Mefloquine
Meloxicam
Mesalamine
Mesoridazine
Methotrexate
Methysergide
Metolazone
Metoprolol
Mexiletine
Mifepristone
Minoxidil
Modafinil
Moexipril
Monosodium glutamate
Moricizine
Moxifloxacin
Nabumetone
Nadolol
Nafarelin
Nalidixic acid
Naltrexone
Naproxen
Naratriptan
Natalizumab
Nedocromil
Nefazodone
Nicotine
Nisoldipine
Nitisinone
Nitrofurantoin
Norfloxacin
Octreotide
Ofloxacin
Olmesartan
Omeprazole
Oxaliplatin

Oxaprozin
Oxcarbazepine
Palonosetron
Pamidronate
Pantoprazole
Paramethadione
Paroxetine
Peginterferon alfa-2B
Pegaptanib
Pegvisomant
Pemetrexed (38–49%)
Penbutolol
Pentamidine
Pentostatin
Pentoxifylline
Pergolide
Perindopril
Perphenazine
Phendimetrazine
Phenelzine
Phenindamine
Phentermine
Pilocarpine
Pindolol
Pioglitazone
Pirbuterol
Piroxicam
Pramipexole
Pravastatin
Praziquantel
Procarbazine
Prochlorperazine
Promazine
Promethazine
Propantheline
Propranolol
Quinapril
Quinethazone
Quinidine
Quinupristin/Dalfopristin
Raloxifene
Ramipril
Rasburicase
Repaglinide

Reserpine
Reteplase
Ribavirin
Rifabutin
Risedronate
Risperidone
Ritodrine
Rizatriptan
Ropinirole
Rosiglitazone
Rosuvastatin
Salmeterol
Sargramostin
Selegiline
Sildenafil
Sirolimus
Smallpox vaccine
Sodium cromoglycate
Sotalol
Stavudine
Streptokinase
Sulfadoxine
Sulfasalazine
Sumatriptan
Tacrolimus
Tadalafil
Tamoxifen
Telithromycin
Tenecteplase
Terbutaline
Thioguanine
Tinidazole
Tinzaparin
Tiopronin
Tiotropium
Tocainide
Tolterodine
Topiramate
Toremifene
Travoprost
Trazodone
Trimipramine
Vasopressin
Verapamil

Vinorelbine
Voriconazole
Zaleplon
Zidovudine
Ziprasidone
Zoledronic acid
Zolmitriptan
Zolpidem

CHILLS
Aldesleukin (>10%)
Alefacept (6%)
Alglucerase
Allopurinol IV
Amifostine
Amphotericin B
Ampicillin
Anagrelide
Anthrax vaccine
Aripiprazole
Asparaginase
Balsalazide
Benzonatate
Bexarotene (10-13%)
Bicalutamide
Botulinum toxin (a & b)
Caspofungin (14%)
Cefaclor
Ceftriaxone
Cefuroxime
Cevimeline
Cidofovir (22%)
Ciprofloxacin
Cladribine
Clofibrate
Clopidogrel
Clozapine
Cocaine
Cyclophosphamide
Cyclosporine
Cytarabine
Dacarbazine
Dactinomycin
Danazol

Darbepoetin alfa
Daunorubicin
Denileukin (81%)
Desmopressin
Dicumarol
Didanosine
Dinoprostone
Disopyramide
Docetaxel
Dofetilide
Dolasetron
Doxazosin
Doxorubicin
Efalizumab (13%)
Efavirenz
Enfuvirtide
Enoxaparin
Entacapone
Ephedrine
Epinephrine
Eplerenone
Escitalopram
Esomeprazole
Estramustine
Etanercept
Ethacrynic acid
Ethchlorvynol
Ethosuximide
Ethotoin
Etoposide
Exemestane
Ezetimibe
Fenofibrate
Floxuridine
Fluconazole
Fludarabine
Fluorouracil
Fluoxetine
Fluoxymesterone
Flurazepam
Flurbiprofen
Flutamide
Fondaparinux
Fosinopril

Fosphenytoin
Fulvestrant
Furosemide
Gabapentin
Gatifloxacin
Gefitinib
Gemcitabine
Gemfibrozil
Gemifloxacin
Gemtuzumab (66%)
Glatiramer
Gold
Goserelin
Heparin
Hepatitis B vaccine
Hydralazine
Hydrochlorothiazide
Hydroflumethiazide
Hydroxyurea
Ibandronate
Ibritumomab (24%)
Ifosfamide
Imatinib
Immune globulin IV
Influenza vaccines
Interferon alfa-2A
Interferon beta-1A (20%)
Interferon beta-1B (25%)
Itraconazole
Ketoconazole
Ketoprofen
Lamivudine
Lamotrigine
Laronidase
Leflunomide
Letrozole
Levalbuterol
Levamisole
Levodopa
Levofloxacin
Lomustine
Lomefloxacin
Lovastatin
Mechlorethamine

Meclofenamate
Medroxyprogesterone
Mefenamic acid
Mefloquine
Melphalan
Mephenytoin
Meprobamate
Mercaptopurine
Mesalamine
Metformin
Methotrexate
Methsuximide
Methyclothiazide
Methyldopa
Methyltestosterone
Methysergide
Metoclopramide
Metolazone
Mexiletine
Midodrine
Mifepristone
Mirtazapine
Mitomycin
Mitoxantrone
Modafinil
Moxifloxacin
Nalidixic acid
Naltrexone
Naratriptan
Nateglinide
Nefazodone
Nelfinavir
Niacin
Nifedipine
Nitisinone
Nitrofurantoin
Norfloxacin
Ofloxacin
Olmesartan
Omalizumab
Oxcarbazepine
Paclitaxel
Palonosetron
Pamidronate

Paricalcitol
Paroxetine
Peginterferon alfa-2B
Pegvisomant
Pemetrexed
Pemirolast
Pentagastrin
Pentamidine
Pentazocine
Pentosan
Pentostatin (>10%)
Pergolide
Phenytoin
Pilocarpine
Polythiazide
Pravastatin
Probenecid
Procainamide
Propantheline
Propofol
Propoxyphene
Quetiapine
Quinine
Rabeprazole
Rasburicase
Repaglinide
Reteplase
Rifabutin
Rifampin
Riluzole
Risperidone
Ritonavir
Rituximab (33%)
Rizatriptan
Ropinirole
Rosiglitazone
Sibutramine
Sirolimus
Spectinomycin
Stavudine
Streptokinase
Streptozocin
Sulfadoxine
Sulfasalazine

Tacrolimus
Tegaserod
Telithromycin
Thiabendazole
Thioguanine
Thiotepa
Tiagabine
Ticarcillin
Tinidazole
Tinzaparin
Tiopronin
Tiotropium
Tizanidine
Topiramate
Topotecan
Trandolapril
Tranylcypromine
Trastuzumab
Travoprost
Trazodone
Trimethoprim
Unoprostone
Urofollitropin
Valdecoxib
Valganciclovir
Vancomycin
Vinblastine
Vinorelbine
Voriconazole
Warfarin
Zalcitabine
Zaleplon
Zidovudine
Ziprasidone
Zoledronic acid
Zolmitriptan
Zonisamide

CHOREOATHETOSIS
Citalopram

CHRONIC FATIGUE SYNDROME
Anthrax vaccine
Fluorides

COMA
Abciximab (<1%)
Acyclovir
Aldesleukin (2%)
Alemtuzumab
Allopurinol IV
Amantadine
Amitriptyline
Amphotericin B
Arsenic
Asparaginase
Aspirin
Bortezomib
Carmustine
Cefepime
Ceftazidime
Cevimeline
Clonazepam
Clozapine
Cycloserine
Daptomycin
Desmopressin
Dicyclomine
Diethylpropion
Escitalopram
Fluphenazine
Gabapentin
Glatiramer
Glycopyrrolate
Hydralazine
Interferon alfa-2A
Lamotrigine
Lidocaine
Lithium
Lomefloxacin
Mazindol
Mesoridazine
Methotrexate
Moxifloxacin
Nitisinone
Paramethadione
Paroxetine
Pemoline
Perphenazine

Phendimetrazine
Phentermine
Pimozide
Prochlorperazine
Promazine
Promethazine
Propantheline
Rabeprazole
Rasburicase
Reteplase
Rosiglitazone
Streptokinase
Thimerosal
Trimetrexate

DEAFNESS
Celecoxib
Mechlorethamine
Salsalate
Sirolimus
Streptomycin

DEATH
Celecoxib
Chloral hydrate
Chlormezanone
Chlorpromazine
Chlorpropamide
Cimetidine
Ciprofloxacin
Citalopram
Clonazepam
Clozapine
Colchicine
Collagen
Comfrey
Cyclosporine
Dacarbazine
Danazol
Daunorubicin
Desflurane
Desmopressin
Diclofenac
Dicyclomine

Didanosine
Diphenhydramine
Docetaxel
Domperidone
Doxorubicin
Enalapril
Etanercept
Ethchlorvynol
Fentanyl
Fludarabine
Fluorides
Fluorouracil
Fluvastatin
Furosemide
Gemcitabine
Gemfibrozil
Glycopyrrolate
Goldenseal
Granulocyte colony-stimulating factor
(GCSF)
Griseofulvin
Guarana
Haloperidol
Hepatitis B vaccine
Hydralazine
Hydroxychloroquine
Hydroxyurea
Ibritumomab
Ibuprofen
Ifosfamide
Imatinib
Immune globulin IV
Indomethacin
Infliximab
Interferon beta-1A
Ipratropium
Irinotecan
Isoniazid
Isotretinoin
Itraconazole
Kava
Ketoconazole
Lamotrigine
Leflunomide

Leucovorin
Levofloxacin
Lidocaine
Lindane
Lomefloxacin
Lovastatin
Mafenide
MDMA
Mefloquine
Melphalan
Metformin
Methadone
Methamphetamine
Methotrexate
Morphine
Moxifloxacin
Nalbuphine
Naltrexone
Naproxen
Nefazodone
Nelfinavir
Nitisinone
Nitrofurantoin
Norfloxacin
Ofloxacin
Olanzapine
Oxaliplatin
Oxaprozin
Oxycodone
Paclitaxel
Pemetrexed
Penicillamine
Penicillins
Phenobarbital
Phenylpropanolamine
Phenytoin
Physostigmine
Pimozide
Pravastatin
Propantheline
Propofol
Propoxyphene
Protamine sulfate
Protriptyline

Pyrazinamide
Pyrimethamine
Rifampin
Risperidone
Rituximab
Rue
Smallpox vaccine
Stanozolol
Thimerosal
Zidovudine

DIPLOPIA

Baclofen
Sirolimus
Streptokinase
Telithromycin
Timolol
Tiopronin
Topiramate
Unoprostone
Vigabatrin
Vinblastine

DIZZINESS

Abarelix (12%)
Acamprosate (3%)
Acebutolol (6%)
Acetazolamide
Acetohexamide
Acetylcysteine
Acitretin (<1%)
Acyclovir (1–10%)
Adenosine (1–10%)
Agalsidase (14%)
Albendazole (1–10%)
Albuterol
Aldesleukin (11%)
Alefacept (1–10%)
Alfuzosin (6%)
Almotriptan (>1%)
Alemtuzumab (12%)
Alprazolam (2–30%)
Alprostadil (2–10%)
Altretamine (<1%)

Amantadine (5–10%)
Amifostine
Amiloride
Aminocaproic acid
Aminophylline
Amiodarone
Amitriptyline
Amlodipine
Amoxapine
Amoxicillin
Amphotericin B
Anastrozole
Anthrax vaccine
Apomorphine·
Apraclonidine
Aprepitant
Aprotinin
Aripiprazole
Arsenic
Ascorbic acid
Aspirin
Atazanavir
Atenolol
Atomoxetine
Azacitidine
Azithromycin
Aztreonam
Baclofen
Balsalazide
Basiliximab
Benazepril
Bendroflumethiazide
Benzonatate
Benzphetamine
Benztropine
Bepridil
Betaxolol
Bevacizumab
Bexarotene
Bicalutamide
Black cohosh
Bortezomib (21%)
Botulinum toxin (a & b)
Bretylium

Brinzolamide
Bromocriptine (17%)
Bumetanide
Bupropion
Buspirone (12%)
Cabergoline (17%)
Calcitonin
Carbinoxamine
Candesartan
Capecitabine
Capreomycin
Carbamazepine (>10%)
Carbinoxamine
Carisoprodol
Carmustine
Carteolol
Carvedilol (32%)
Cascara
Caspofungin
Cefaclor
Cefdinir
Cefditoren
Cefixime
Ceftazidime
Ceftibuten
Ceftriaxone
Cefuroxime
Celecoxib
Cephalexin
Cephradine
Cetirizine
Cevimeline
Chloral hydrate
Chlordiazepoxide (1–10%)
Chlorothiazide
Chlorotrianisene
Chlorpromazine
Chlorpropamide
Chlorthalidone
Chlorzoxazone
Cilostazol (10%)
Cimetidine
Cinacalcet (10%)
Cinoxacin

Ciprofloxacin
Citalopram
Cladribine
Clarithromycin
Clemastine
Clofarabine (16%)
Clofazimine
Clomiphene
Clomipramine (>10%)
Clonazepam (>10%)
Clonidine (16%)
Clopidogrel
Clorazepate
Clozapine (>10%)
Cocaine
Codeine
Colestipol
Corticosteroids
Cyanocobalamin
Cyclobenzaprine (11%)
Cyclophosphamide
Cycloserine
Cyproheptadine
Cytarabine
Dacarbazine
Daclizumab
Dalteparin
Danaparoid
Dantrolene
Daptomycin
Darbepoetin alfa
Delavirdine
Denileukin (22%)
Desflurane
Desipramine
Desloratadine
Desmopressin
Dextroamphetamine
Dextromethorphan
Diazepam
Diclofenac
Dicloxacillin
Dicumarol
Dicyclomine

Diethylpropion
Diflunisal
Digoxin
Dihydroergotamine
Diltiazem
Dimenhydrinate
Dinoprostone
Diphenhydramine
Diphenoxylate
Dipyridamole (14%)
Dirithromycin
Disopyramide
Dobutamine
Docetaxel
Docusate
Dofetilide
Dolasetron
Domperidone
Donepezil
Dorzolamide
Doxazosin (>16–19%)
Doxepin
Doxercalciferol (12%)
Doxorubicin
Doxycycline
Dronabinol (21%)
Duloxetine (10%)
Dutasteride
Echinacea
Edrophonium
Efavirenz (2–28%)
Eflornithine
Eletriptan
Emtricitabine (25%)
Enalapril
Enflurane
Enfuvirtide
Enoxaparin
Entacapone
Ephedrine
Epinephrine
Eplerenone
Epoetin alfa
Eprosartan

Ertapenem
Escitalopram
Esmolol
Esomeprazole
Estazolam
Estrogens
Etanercept
Ethacrynic acid
Ethambutol
Ethchlorvynol
Ethionamide
Ethosuximide
Ethotoin
Etodolac
Eucalyptus
Exemestane
Ezetimibe
Famciclovir
Famotidine
Felbamate
Felodipine
Fenofibrate
Fenoldopam
Fenoprofen (7–15%)
Fentanyl
Fexofenadine
Finasteride
Flavoxate
Flecainide (19%)
Floxuridine
Fluconazole
Flucytosine
Fludarabine
Flumazenil
Fluoxetine
Fluoxymesterone
Flurazepam
Flurbiprofen
Flutamide
Fluvastatin
Fluvoxamine
Fomepizole
Fondaparinux
Formoterol

Foscarnet
Fosfomycin
Fosinopril (2–12%)
Fosphenytoin (<10%)
Frovatriptan
Fulvestrant
Furosemide
Gabapentin (17%)
Gadodiamide
Galantamine
Gatifloxacin
Gemcitabine
Gemfibrozil
Gemifloxacin
Gemtuzumab (11%)
Gentamicin
Glatiramer
Glimepiride
Glipizide
Glucagon
Glyburide
Glycopyrrolate
Goserelin
Granisetron
Granulocyte colony-stimulating factor
(GCSF)
Griseofulvin
Guanabenz
Guanadrel
Guanethidine
Guanfacine
Guarana
Haloperidol
Halothane
Hawthorn (fruit, leaf, flower extract)
Heparin
Hepatitis B vaccine
Hyaluronic acid
Hydralazine
Hydrochlorothiazide
Hydrocodone
Hydroflumethiazide
Hydromorphone
Hydroxychloroquine

Hydroxyurea
Hyoscyamine
Ibandronate
Ibritumomab
Imiglucerase
Imipenem/Cilastatin
Imipramine
Imiquimod
Immune globulin IV
Inamrinone
Indapamide
Indinavir
Indomethacin
Infliximab
Influenza vaccines
Interferon alfa-2A (21%)
Interferon beta-1A (15%)
Interferon beta-1B (24%)
Ipodate
Ipratropium
Irbesartan (10%)
Irinotecan (10%)
Isocarboxazid
Isoetharine
Isoflurane
Isoniazid
Isosorbide dinitrate
Isosorbide mononitrate
Isotretinoin
Isoxsuprine
Isradipine
Itraconazole
Ivermectin
Kava
Ketamine
Ketoconazole
Ketoprofen
Ketorolac
Labetalol (<16%)
Lamivudine
Lamotrigine (38%)
Lansoprazole
Laronidase
Leflunomide

Letrozole
Levalbuterol
Levamisole
Levetiracetam (9–18%)
Levobetaxolol
Levobunolol
Levodopa
Levofloxacin
Lidocaine
Lindane
Linezolid
Lisinopril
Lithium
Lomefloxacin
Loperamide
Loracarbef
Loratadine
Lorazepam
Losartan
Lovastatin
Loxapine
Maprotiline
Mazindol
Mebendazole
Mecamylamine
Mechlorethamine
Meclizine
Meclofenamate
Medroxyprogesterone
Mefenamic acid
Mefloquine
Meloxicam
Memantine
Mepenzolate
Meperidine
Mephenytoin (<10%)
Mephobarbital
Meprobamate
Mesalamine
Metaxalone
Metformin
Methadone
Methamphetamine
Methantheline

Methazolamide
Methicillin
Methimazole
Methocarbamol
Methohexital
Methotrexate
Methoxsalen
Methoxyflurane
Methsuximide
Methyclothiazide
Methyldopa
Methylphenidate
Methyltestosterone
Methysergide
Metipranolol
Metolazone (>10%)
Metoprolol
Metronidazole
Mexiletine (20–25%)
Mezlocillin
Midodrine
Mifepristone (<12%)
Miglustat (<11%)
Minocycline
Mirtazapine
Mitotane (15%)
Modafinil
Modafinil
Molindone
Montelukast
Moricizine (>10%)
Morphine
Moxifloxacin
Mupirocin
Mycophenolate
Nabumetone (>10%)
Nadolol (<16%)
Nafcillin
Nalbuphine
Nalidixic acid
Naltrexone
Naproxen
Naratriptan
Natalizumab

Nateglinide
Nedocromil
Nefazodone (>10%)
Nelfinavir
Nesiritide
Nicardipine
Nicotine
Nifedipine (10–27%)
Nisoldipine
Nitazoxanide
Nitisinone
Nitrofurantoin
Nitroglycerin
Nizatidine
Norfloxacin
Nortriptyline
Octreotide
Ofloxacin
Olanzapine (>10%)
Olmesartan
Olsalazine
Omalizumab
Omeprazole
Ondansetron
Orphenadrine
Oxacillin
Oxaliplatin
Oxaprozin
Oxazepam
Oxcarbazepine (22–44%)
Oxybutynin (6–16%)
Oxycodone (>10%)
Oxytetracycline
Paclitaxel
Palonosetron
Pamidronate
Pantoprazole
Papaverine
Paramethadione
Paricalcitol
Paromomycin
Paroxetine (>10%)
Peginterferon alfa-2B (12%)
Pegaptanib

Pegvisomant
Pemetrexed
Pemoline
Penbutolol (<16%)
Penicillins
Pentagastrin
Pentazocine
Pentobarbital
Pentosan
Pentostatin
Pentoxifylline
Perflutren
Pergolide (19%)
Perindopril
Perphenazine
Phenazopyridine
Phendimetrazine
Phenelzine
Phenindamine
Phenobarbital
Phenoxybenzamine
Phentermine
Phentolamine
Phenylephrine
Phenytoin
Phytonadione
Pilocarpine
Pimozide
Pindolol
Piperacillin
Pirbuterol
Piroxicam (>10%)
Polythiazide
Pramipexole (>10%)
Pravastatin
Prazepam
Praziquantel
Prazosin (>10%)
Primaquine
Primidone
Probenecid
Procainamide
Procarbazine (>10%)
Prochlorperazine

Procyclidine
Progestins
Promazine
Promethazine
Propantheline (4–15%)
Propofol
Propoxyphene
Propranolol (<16%)
Propylthiouracil
Protriptyline
Pseudoephedrine
Pyrimethamine
Quazepam
Quetiapine (>10%)
Quinapril
Quinethazone
Quinidine (>15%)
Quinine
Rabeprazole
Ramipril
Ranitidine
Rasburicase
Reserpine
Reteplase
Ribavirin
Rifampin
Rifapentine
Rifaximin
Riluzole
Rimantadine
Risedronate
Risperidone (>19%)
Ritodrine
Ritonavir
Rituximab (>10%)
Rivastigmine (21%)
Rizatriptan
Rofecoxib
Ropinirole (40%)
Rosuvastatin
Salmeterol
Salsalate
Sargramostin
Scopolamine

Secretin
Selegiline
Sermorelin
Sertraline
Sibutramine
Sildenafil
Simvastatin
Sirolimus
Sodium oxybate
Solifenacin
Sotalol
Sparfloxacin
Spectinomycin
Spironolactone
St John's wort
Stavudine
Streptokinase
Streptomycin
Succimer
Sulfadiazine
Sulfamethoxazole
Sulindac
Sumatriptan
Tadalafil
Tamsulosin
Tegaserod
Telithromycin
Telmisartan
Temazepam
Tenecteplase
Terazosin
Terbutaline
Teriparatide
Thalidomide
Thiabendazole
Thioguanine
Thiopental
Thioridazine
Thiotepa
Thiothixene
Tiagabine
Ticarcillin
Timolol
Tinidazole

Tinzaparin
Tizanidine
Tocainide
Tolazamide
Tolbutamide
Tolcapone
Tolmetin
Topiramate
Toremifene
Torsemide
Tositumomab & iodine 131
Tramadol
Trandolapril
Travoprost
Trazodone
Treprostinil
Triamterene
Triazolam
Trichlormethiazide
Trimethobenzamide
Trifluoperazine
Trihexyphenidyl
Trimeprazine
Trimetrexate
Trimipramine
Trioxsalen
Tripelennamine
Triptorelin
Trovafloxacin
Ursodiol
Valdecoxib
Valrubicin
Valsartan
Vardenafil
Vasopressin
Venlafaxine
Verapamil
Vigabatrin
Vinblastine
Voriconazole
Zafirlukast
Zalcitabine
Zaleplon
Zanamivir

Zidovudine
Zileuton
Ziprasidone
Zoledronic acid
Zolmitriptan
Zonisamide

DYSESTHESIA

Alemtuzumab (15%)
Alfentanil
Aminolevulinic acid
Amphotericin B
Bortezomib (23%)
Ciprofloxacin
Cyclosporine
Docetaxel
Enalapril
Fentanyl
Frovatriptan
Gemifloxacin
Indinavir
Lisinopril
Moexipril
Omeprazole
Oxaliplatin
Palifermin (12%)
Perindopril
Quinapril
Quinethazone
Ramipril
Stanozolol
Tamoxifen
Telithromycin
Vardenafil
Vincristine

DYSGEUSIA

Alosetron
Alprazolam (<1%)
Amifostine
Amiodarone
Amitriptyline
Amoxapine
Amoxicillin

Amprenavir
Apraclonidine
Aprepitant
Arbutamine
Aripiprazole
Arsenic
Aspirin
Azithromycin
Aztreonam
Bacampicillin
Baclofen
Balsalazide
Benazepril
Benzphetamine
Benzthiazide
Benztropine
Bepridil
Betaxolol
Bevacizumab
Bismuth
Bisoprolol
Bortezomib (13%)
Botulinum toxin (a & b)
Brimonidine
Brinzolamide
Bupropion
Buspirone
Calcitonin
Capecitabine
Captopril
Carbamazepine
Carbenicillin (1–10%)
Carteolol
Cefamandole
Cefditoren
Cefmetazole
Cefpodoxime
Ceftazidime
Ceftibuten
Ceftriaxone
Celecoxib
Cetirizine
Cevimeline
Chloral hydrate

Chloramphenicol
Chlorhexidine (>10%)
Chlormezanone
Cholestyramine
Cidofovir
Cinoxacin
Ciprofloxacin
Cisplatin
Citalopram
Clarithromycin
Clidinium
Clindamycin
Clofazimine
Clomipramine
Clonidine
Clopidogrel
Clotrimazole
Clozapine
Co-Trimoxazole
Cocaine (>10%)
Codeine
Cromolyn
Cyclobenzaprine
Danazol
Dapsone
Daptomycin
Delavirdine
Desipramine (>10%)
Devil's claw
Dextroamphetamine
Diazoxide
Diclofenac
Dicloxacillin
Dicyclomine
Diethylpropion
Dihydroergotamine
Dihydrotachysterol
Dipyridamole
Dirithromycin
Disulfiram
Docetaxel
Docusate
Dolasetron
Dorzolamide (25%)

Doxazosin
Doxepin (>10%)
Doxercalciferol
Doxorubicin
Doxycycline
Dronabinol
Efavirenz
Eletriptan
Enalapril
Enfuvirtide
Enoxacin
Entacapone (20%)
Eprosartan
Ergocalciferol
Escitalopram
Esmolol
Esomeprazole
Estazolam
Estrogens
Etanercept
Ethchlorvynol (>10%)
Ethionamide
Etidronate
Etodolac
Etoposide
Famotidine
Felbamate
Fenoprofen
Fentanyl
Feverfew
Flecainide
Fluconazole
Fludarabine
Fluorouracil
Fluoxetine
Flurazepam
Flurbiprofen
Fluvastatin
Fluvoxamine
Fomepizole
Foscarnet
Fosinopril
Fosphenytoin
Frovatriptan

Gadodiamide
Ganciclovir
Gatifloxacin
Gemcitabine
Gemfibrozil
Gemifloxacin
Glatiramer
Glimepiride
Glipizide
Glyburide
Glycopyrrolate
Gold
Granisetron
Granulocyte colony-stimulating factor (GCSF)
Griseofulvin
Guanfacine
Hydrochlorothiazide
Hydrocodone
Hydroflumethiazide
Hydroxychloroquine
Hyoscyamine
Ibuprofen
Imatinib (<14%)
Imipenem/Cilastatin
Imipramine (>10%)
Indinavir
Indomethacin
Interferon alfa-2A (25%)
Interferon beta-1A
Interferon beta-1B
Ipratropium
Isotretinoin
Ketoprofen
Ketorolac
Labetalol
Lamotrigine
Lansoprazole
Leflunomide
Letrozole
Leuprolide
Levamisole
Levobetaxolol
Levobunolol

Levodopa
Levofloxacin
Linezolid
Lisinopril
Lithium (>10%)
Lomefloxacin
Loratadine
Losartan
Lovastatin
Maprotiline
Mazindol
Mechlorethamine
Meclofenamate
Mefenamic acid
Meloxicam
Mepenzolate
Meperidine
Mephenytoin
Mesalamine
Mesna (>17%)
Metformin
Methadone
Methamphetamine
Methantheline
Methazolamide (>10%)
Methicillin
Methimazole
Methocarbamol
Methotrexate
Methyclothiazide
Metipranolol
Metolazone
Metoprolol
Metronidazole
Mezlocillin
Midazolam
Minocycline
Minoxidil
Mirtazapine
Misoprostol
Modafinil
Moexipril
Moricizine
Morphine

Moxifloxacin
Mupirocin
Nabumetone
Nadolol
Nafcillin
Nalbuphine
Naproxen
Naratriptan
Nedocromil (<12%)
Nefazodone
Nicotine
Nizatidine
Norfloxacin
Nortriptyline (>10%)
Ofloxacin
Olanzapine
Olopatadine
Omeprazole
Ondansetron
Oxacillin
Oxaliplatin
Oxaprozin
Oxcarbazepine
Oxybutynin
Oxycodone
Oxytetracycline
Palifermin (16%)
Pantoprazole
Paricalcitol
Paroxetine
Peginterferon alfa-2B
Pegfilgrastim
Penbutolol
Penicillamine (12%)
Penicillins
Pentamidine
Pentazocine
Pentostatin
Pentoxifylline
Pergolide
Perindopril
Phendimetrazine
Phenindamine
Phentermine

Phenytoin
Phytonadione
Pilocarpine
Pimozide
Pindolol
Piperacillin
Pirbuterol
Piroxicam
Plicamycin
Polythiazide
Potassium iodide
Pramipexole
Pravastatin
Procainamide
Propantheline (3–23%)
Propofol
Propoxyphene
Propranolol
Propylthiouracil
Protriptyline (>10%)
Pyrimethamine
Quazepam
Quinethazone
Quinidine (>10%)
Ramipril
Ranitidine
Ribavirin
Rifabutin
Rimantadine
Risperidone
Ritonavir (>10%)
Rivastigmine
Saquinavir
Scopolamine (29%)
Secobarbital
Sibutramine
Sparfloxacin
Telithromycin
Terbinafine
Tinidazole
Tiopronin
Trazodone
Triazolam
Trimethadione

Valrubicin
Zalcitabine
Zaleplon
Zidovudine (5–19%)
Zolpidem (<1%)
Zonisamide (2%)

DYSKINESIA

Allopurinol IV
Amitriptyline
Apomorphine
Aripiprazole
Aripiprazole
Baclofen
Bupropion
Cabergoline
Carbamazepine
Ceftazidime
Cetirizine
Cevimeline
Chlorambucil
Chlorpromazine
Citalopram
Clomipramine (>10%)
Clonazepam (>10%)
Cocaine
Diltiazem
Droperidol
Entacapone (31%)
Estrogens
Felbamate
Fluoxetine
Fluphenazine
Frovatriptan
Gabapentin
Haloperidol
Levodopa
Lithium
Loxapine
Mecamylamine
Mephenytoin
Mesoridazine
Methocarbamol
Methylphenidate

Modafinil
Molindone
Moxifloxacin
Nitazoxanide
Olanzapine
Ondansetron
Oxcarbazepine
Paroxetine
Pemetrexed
Pergolide (12%)
Perphenazine
Phenelzine
Pimozide
Pramipexole (>10%)
Prochlorperazine
Promazine
Promethazine
Propofol
Propranolol
Protriptyline
Quinidine
Rasburicase
Risperidone
Rizatriptan
Ropinirole
Sirolimus
Tiagabine
Tizanidine
Tolazamide
Topiramate
Trifluoperazine
Trimethadione
Trimethobenzamide
Trimipramine

DYSPHAGIA

Ezetimibe
Hyaluronic acid
Hyoscyamine
Interferon beta-1A
Irinotecan
Itraconazole
Ketoconazole
Ketoprofen

Lamotrigine
Leuprolide
Levodopa
Meclofenamate
Mefenamic acid
Meloxicam
Melphalan
Mepenzolate
Methantheline
Molindone
Nabumetone
Olanzapine
Olmesartan
Omalizumab
Oxaliplatin
Oxaprozin
Oxcarbazepine
Paroxetine
Pemetrexed
Pentosan
Pentoxifylline
Pergolide
Phenytoin
Phytonadione
Pilocarpine
Pimozide
Pramipexole
Procarbazine (>10%)
Procyclidine
Propantheline
Quetiapine
Quinine
Rabeprazole
Ramipril
Rasburicase
Riluzole
Risperidone
Ritonavir
Rizatriptan
Ropinirole
Rosuvastatin
Salmeterol
Sirolimus
Stavudine

Sulfadiazine
Sulfamethoxazole
Sulfasalazine
Tenecteplase
Tinidazole
Tizanidine
Topiramate
Trandolapril
Tranylcypromine
Triazolam
Trimethadione
Trimethoprim
Trimipramine
Trovafloxacin

DYSPHASIA

Capecitabine
Donepezil
Glatiramer
Ibuprofen
Paroxetine
Piroxicam
Propantheline
Sermorelin
Tiagabine
Tizanidine
Topiramate
Trimethobenzamide
Trimipramine
Vigabatrin

DYSPHONIA

Balsalazide
Cetirizine
Edrophonium
Estrogens
Etanercept
Etodolac
Formoterol
Mepenzolate
Propoxyphene
Rivastigmine
Vancomycin

Zalcitabine
Zonisamide

EAR PAIN
Aripiprazole
Arsenic
Balsalazide
Calcitonin
Cefaclor
Celecoxib
Cetirizine
Cevimeline
Cisplatin
Dipyridamole
Fenofibrate
Frovatriptan
Gatifloxacin
Glatiramer
Hepatitis B vaccine
Isotretinoin
Levalbuterol
Levofloxacin
Lomefloxacin
Moxifloxacin
Nefazodone
Nitisinone
Norfloxacin
Ofloxacin
Orlistat
Pentostatin
Pimecrolimus
Salmeterol
Sirolimus
Streptomycin
Zanamivir

ENCEPHALOPATHY
Adenosine (<1%)
Albendazole (1%)
Amiloride
Aminosalicylic acid
Ampicillin
Aripiprazole
Aspirin

Bumetanide
Capecitabine
Carmustine (23%)
Cefepime
Ceftazidime
Chlorpromazine
Fosphenytoin
Gabapentin
Ganciclovir
Gemfibrozil
Gemtuzumab
Levofloxacin
Lomefloxacin
Mefloquine
Methotrexate
Mephenytoin
Moxifloxacin
Nalidixic acid
Nitisinone
Norfloxacin
Ofloxacin
Paclitaxel
Pentazocine
Phenytoin
Propoxyphene
Quinupristin/Dalfopristin
Streptomycin

EXTRAPYRAMIDAL SYNDROME
Amitriptyline
Aripiprazole
Desipramine
Doxepin
Droperidol
Fosphenytoin
Imipramine
Ketorolac
Mephenytoin
Metoclopramide
Nortriptyline
Ondansetron
Oxcarbazepine
Phenytoin
Pramipexole

Protriptyline
Risperidone (>10%)

EYE PAIN
Aripiprazole
Bimatoprost
Carmustine
Celecoxib
Cetirizine
Cevimeline
Ciprofloxacin
Citalopram
Clidinium
Clomipramine
Clonazepam
Corticosteroids
Danazol
Disulfiram
Estrogens
Etanercept
Etodolac
Flavoxate
Fluoxetine
Flurbiprofen
Frovatriptan
Hyoscyamine
Ibandronate
Ibuprofen
Indomethacin
Isoniazid
Ivermectin
Ketoprofen
Ketotifen
Latanoprost
Lithium
Meclofenamate
Mefenamic acid
Mepenzolate
Methantheline
Modafinil
Naproxen
Nefazodone
Nitisinone
Olopatadine

Orphenadrine
Oxybutynin
Pamidronate
Paroxetine
Pegaptanib
Physostigmine
Piroxicam
Procyclidine
Propantheline
Sirolimus
Sulfacetamide
Tacrolimus
Tiotropium
Tizanidine
Topiramate
Travoprost
Trihexyphenidyl
Unoprostone
Vigabatrin
Voriconazole

FACIAL PAIN
Aripiprazole
Darbepoetin alfa
Zanamivir

FACIAL PALSY
Anthrax vaccine
Lovastatin
Zalcitabine

GUILLAIN-BARRE SYNDROME
Norfloxacin

GLOSSITIS
Balsalazide
Carbenicillin (1–10%)
Ceftazidime
Ceftriaxone
Chloramphenicol
Chlorhexidine
Citalopram
Clarithromycin
Cloxacillin

Co-Trimoxazole
Cyclosporine
Dicloxacillin
Doxorubicin
Doxycycline
Enalapril
Estazolam
Etidronate
Felbamate
Fenoprofen
Floxuridine
Fluoxetine
Fluvoxamine
Gabapentin
Gatifloxacin
Gold
Guanadrel
Guanfacine
Hydroxyurea
Imipenem/Cilastatin
Imipramine
Interferon beta-1A
Interferon beta-1B
Lansoprazole
Levodopa
Levofloxacin
Lincomycin
Lomefloxacin
Mecamylamine
Mefenamic acid
Mercaptopurine
Methadone
Methicillin
Methotrexate
Metronidazole
Mezlocillin
Minocycline
Mirtazapine
Morphine
Moxifloxacin
Nabumetone
Nafcillin
Nalbuphine
Nefazodone

Nisoldipine
Norfloxacin
Nortriptyline
Ofloxacin
Oxacillin
Oxytetracycline
Pantoprazole
Paroxetine
Penicillamine
Peppermint
Phenelzine
Pilocarpine
Piperacillin
Pirbuterol
Protriptyline
Pyrimethamine
Quetiapine
Rabeprazole
Risedronate
Rivastigmine
Ropinirole
Zalcitabine
Zonisamide (<1%)

GLOSSODYNIA

Bacampicillin
Biperiden
Cloxacillin
Clozapine
Dicloxacillin
Doxepin
Erythromycin
Etodolac
Fluoxetine
Glatiramer
Griseofulvin
Ibuprofen
Imipramine
Indomethacin
Lithium
Methicillin
Methyldopa
Mezlocillin
Nafcillin

Naproxen
Nortriptyline
Olanzapine
Oxacillin
Oxaprozin
Piperacillin
Piroxicam
Protriptyline
Rifampin
Zalcitabine

HEADACHE

Abacavir (16%)
Abarelix (12%)
Abciximab (6%)
Acebutolol (6%)
Acetaminophen
Acetazolamide
Acitretin (10%)
Acyclovir (1–10%)
Abacavir
Abarelix
Abciximab
Acamprosate
Acetaminophen
Acetazolamide
Acetohexamide
Acyclovir
Adalimumab (12%)
Adefovir (1–10%)
Adenosine (>10%)
Agalsidase (45%)
Albendazole (11%)
Albuterol
Aldesleukin
Alefacept (<1%)
Alemtuzumab (24%)
Alendronate (>3%)
Alfuzosin (3%)
Alglucerase
Alitretinoin
Allopurinol
Almotriptan (>1%)
Alprazolam (13–30%)

Alprostadil (2–10%
Alteplase
Amantadine (1–5%)
Amiloride
Aminocaproic acid
Aminoglutethimide
Aminophylline
Amiodarone
Amitriptyline
Amlodipine
Amobarbital
Amoxapine
Amoxicillin
Amphotericin B
Ampicillin
Amprenavir
Amyl nitrite
Anagrelide
Anakinra
Anastrozole
Androstenedione
Anthrax vaccine
Apomorphine
Apraclonidine
Aprepitant
Argatroban
Aripiprazole
Arsenic
Ascorbic acid
Asparaginase
Aspirin
Atazanavir
Atomoxetine
Atorvastatin
Atovaquone
Atropine sulfate
Azacitidine
Azelastine
Azithromycin
Aztreonam
Baclofen
Balsalazide
Basiliximab
Benazepril

Bendroflumethiazide
Benzonatate
Benzphetamine
Bepridil
Betaxolol
Bethanechol
Bevacizumab
Bexarotene (30–42%)
Bicalutamide
Bimatoprost
Bismuth
Bisoprolol
Bivalirudin
Bortezomib (28%)
Bosentan (22%)
Botulinum toxin (a & b) (11%)
Brimonidine
Brinzolamide
Bromocriptine (19%)
Brompheniramine
Buclizine
Bumetanide
Bupropion
Buspirone
Busulfan
Butalbital
Butorphanol
Cabergoline (26%)
Caffeine
Calcitonin
Candesartan
Capecitabine (10%)
Captopril
Carbachol
Carbamazepine
Carbenicillin
Carbinoxamine
Carisoprodol
Carmustine (28%)
Carteolol
Carvedilol
Caspofungin (11%)
Cefaclor
Cefdinir

Cefditoren
Cefepime
Cefixime
Cefmetazole
Cefotaxime
Cefpodoxime
Cefprozil
Ceftazidime
Ceftibuten
Ceftriaxone
Cefuroxime
Celecoxib (16%)
Cephalexin
Cetirizine
Cetrorelix
Cetuximab (14%)
Cevimeline
Chasteberry
Chloral hydrate
Chloramphenicol
Chlordiazepoxide
Chloroquine
Chlorotrianisene
Chlorpromazine
Chlorpropamide
Chlorthalidone
Cholestyramine
Cidofovir (30%)
Cilostazol (27–34%)
Cimetidine
Cinoxacin
Ciprofloxacin
Citalopram
Cladribine (22%)
Clarithromycin
Clemastine
Clofarabine (46%)
Clofazimine
Clomiphene
Clomipramine (>10%)
Clonazepam (>10%)
Clonidine
Clopidogrel
Clorazepate

Clotrimazole
Clozapine
Codeine
Co-Trimoxazole
Cocaine
Codeine
Colchicine
Corticosteroids
Cromolyn
Cyanocobalamin
Cyclobenzaprine
Cyclophosphamide
Cycloserine
Cyclosporine
Cyproheptadine
Cytarabine
Dacarbazine
Daclizumab
Dalteparin
Danaparoid
Danazol
Dantrolene
Dapsone
Daptomycin
Darbepoetin alfa
Daunorubicin
Delavirdine
Demeclocycline
Denileukin (26%)
Desflurane
Desipramine
Desloratadine (>10%)
Desmopressin
Dexchlorpheniramine
Dextroamphetamine
Dextromethorphan
Diazepam
Diazoxide
Diclofenac
Dicumarol
Dicloxacillin
Dicyclomine
Didanosine
Diethylpropion

Diflunisal
Digoxin
Dihydroergotamine
Dihydrotachysterol
Diltiazem
Dimenhydrinate
Dimercaprol
Dinoprostone
Diphenhydramine
Diphenoxylate
Dipyridamole
Dirithromycin
Disopyramide
Disulfiram
Dobutamine
Docetaxel
Docosanol
Dofetilide (11%)
Dolasetron (24%)
Domperidone
Donepezil (>10%)
Dopamine
Dorzolamide
Doxazosin (10–14%)
Doxepin
Doxercalciferol (28%)
Doxorubicin
Doxycycline
Dronabinol
Duloxetine (15%)
Edrophonium
Efalizumab (32%)
Efavirenz
Eflornithine
Eletriptan
Emtricitabine (16%)
Enalapril
Enflurane
Enfuvirtide
Enoxaparin
Entacapone
Ephedrine
Epinastine (10%)
Epinephrine

Eplerenone
Epoetin alfa
Ergocalciferol
Ertapenem
Erythromycin
Escitalopram
Esmolol
Esomeprazole
Estazolam
Estrogens
Etanercept (17%)
Ethambutol
Ethionamide
Ethosuximide
Ethotoin
Etodolac
Exemestane
Ezetimibe
Famciclovir
Famotidine
Felbamate
Felodipine (11–15%)
Fenofibrate
Fenoldopam
Fenoprofen
Fentanyl
Fexofenadine (7–11%)
Finasteride
Flavoxate
Flecainide
Fluconazole
Flucytosine
Flumazenil
Fluorides
Fluorouracil
Fluoxetine (21%)
Fluphenazine
Flurazepam
Flurbiprofen
Flutamide
Fluvastatin
Fluvoxamine (>10%)
Fomepizole (14%)
Fondaparinux

Formoterol
Fosamprenavir (20%)
Foscarnet (>10%)
Fosfomycin (47%)
Fosinopril
Fosphenytoin
Frovatriptan
Fulvestrant (15%)
Furazolidone
Furosemide
Gabapentin
Gadodiamide
Galantamine
Ganciclovir
Ganirelix
Gatifloxacin
Gemcitabine
Gemfibrozil
Gemifloxacin
Gemtuzumab (37%)
Gentamicin
Glatiramer
Glimepiride
Glipizide
Glucagon
Glyburide
Glycopyrrolate
Gold and gold compounds
Goserelin (5–75%)
Granisetron (8–21%)
Granulocyte colony-stimulating factor
(GCSF) (39–80%)
Grapefruit juice
Griseofulvin
Guanabenz
Guanadrel
Guanethidine
Guanfacine
Haloperidol
Halothane
Heparin
Hepatitis B vaccine
Hyaluronic acid
Hydralazine

Hydrochlorothiazide
Hydrocodone
Hydroxychloroquine
Hyoscyamine
Hydroxyurea
Hydroxyzine
Hyoscyamine
Ibandronate
Ibritumomab (12%)
Ibuprofen
Ibutilide
Idarubicin
Imatinib (25–35%)
Imiglucerase
Imipramine
Imiquimod
Immune globulin IV
Indapamide
Indinavir
Indomethacin
Infliximab (18%)
Influenza vaccines
Insulin
Interferon alfa-2A (52%)
Interferon beta-1A (>50%)
Interferon beta-1B (57%)
Ipodate
Ipratropium
Irbesartan
Irinotecan
Isocarboxazid
Isoetharine
Isoflurane
Isoniazid
Isoproterenol
Isosorbide dinitrate
Isosorbide mononitrate (19–38%)
Isotretinoin
Isradipine (2–22%)
Itraconazole
Ivermectin
Ketamine
Ketoconazole
Ketoprofen

Ketorolac
Ketotifen
Labetalol
Lamivudine (>10%)
Lamotrigine (29%)
Lansoprazole
Laronidase
Leflunomide
Letrozole (8–12%)
Leuprolide
Levalbuterol
Levamisole
Levetiracetam (24%)
Levobetaxolol
Levobunolol
Levodopa
Levofloxacin
Levothyroxine
Lidocaine
Lindane
Linezolid
Liothyronine
Lisinopril
Lithium
Lomefloxacin
Loracarbef
Loratadine
Lorazepam
Losartan
Lovastatin
Loxapine
Maprotiline
Mazindol
Mebendazole
Mechlorethamine
Meclizine
Meclofenamate
Medroxyprogesterone
Mefenamic acid
Mefloquine
Meloxicam
Memantine
Mepenzolate
Meperidine

Mephenytoin
Mephobarbital
Meprobamate
Mercaptopurine
Mesalamine (14%)
Mesoridazine
Metaxalone
Metformin
Methadone
Methamphetamine
Methazolamide
Methenamine
Methicillin
Methimazole
Methocarbamol
Methohexital
Methotrexate
Methoxsalen
Methoxyflurane
Methsuximide
Methyldopa
Methylphenidate
Methyltestosterone
Methysergide
Metipranolol
Metoclopramide
Metolazone
Metoprolol
Metronidazole
Mexiletine
Mezlocillin
Miconazole
Midazolam
Midodrine
Mifepristone (2–31%)
Miglustat (21%)
Minocycline
Minoxidil
Mirtazapine
Misoprostol
Mitotane
Mitoxantrone (6–13%)
Modafinil (34%)
Moexipril

Molindone
Monosodium glutamate
Montelukast (18%)
Moricizine
Morphine
Moxifloxacin
Mupirocin
Mycophenolate (16–54%)
Myrrh
Nabumetone
Nadolol
Nafarelin (>10%)
Nafcillin
Nalbuphine
Nalidixic acid
Naloxone
Naltrexone (>10%)
Naproxen
Naratriptan
Natalizumab
Nateglinide
Nedocromil
Nefazodone (>10%)
Nelfinavir
Nesiritide
Nevirapine
Niacin
Nicardipine
Nicotine (<10%)
Nifedipine (10–23%)
Nimodipine
Nisoldipine
Nitazoxanide
Nitrofurantoin
Nitroglycerin (>40%)
Nizatidine (16%)
Norfloxacin
Nortriptyline
Octreotide
Ofloxacin
Olanzapine (>10%)
Olmesartan
Olopatadine
Olsalazine

Omalizumab (15%)
Omeprazole
Ondansetron (9–27%)
Orlistat (31%)
Orphenadrine
Oseltamivir
Oxacillin
Oxaliplatin (13%)
Oxaprozin
Oxazepam
Oxcarbazepine (13–32%)
Oxybutynin (6–10%)
Oxycodone
Palonosetron
Pamidronate
Pantoprazole
Papaverine
Paramethadione
Paromomycin
Paroxetine (>10%)
Peginterferon alfa-2B (56%)
Pegaptanib
Pegfilgrastim
Pemetrexed
Pegvisomant
Pemirolast
Pemoline
Penbutolol
Penicillins
Pentagastrin
Pentamidine
Pentazocine
Pentobarbital
Pentosan
Pentostatin
Pentoxifylline
Perflutren
Pergolide
Perindopril (23%)
Perphenazine
Phenazopyridine
Phendimetrazine
Phenelzine
Phenindamine

Phenobarbital
Phenoxybenzamine
Phentermine
Phenylephrine
Phenytoin
Phytonadione
Pilocarpine (11%)
Pimecrolimus (7–25%)
Pimozide
Pioglitazone
Piperacillin
Pirbuterol
Piroxicam
Plicamycin
Pramipexole
Pravastatin
Prazepam
Praziquantel
Prazosin
Primaquine
Probenecid
Procarbazine (>10%)
Prochlorperazine
Procyclidine
Progestins
Promazine
Promethazine
Propafenone
Propantheline
Propofol
Propoxyphene
Propranolol
Propylthiouracil
Protamine sulfate
Protriptyline
Pseudoephedrine
Pyridoxine
Quazepam
Quetiapine (>10%)
Quinapril
Quinethazone
Quinidine
Quinine
Quinupristin/Dalfopristin

Rabeprazole
Ramipril
Ranitidine (16%)
Rasburicase (26%)
Repaglinide (10%)
Reserpine
Reteplase
Ribavirin (50%)
Rifabutin
Rifampin
Rifapentine
Rifaximin
Riluzole
Rimantadine
Risedronate (18%)
Risperidone (>10%)
Ritodrine
Ritonavir
Rituximab (19%)
Rivastigmine (17%)
Rizatriptan
Rofecoxib
Ropinirole
Rosiglitazone
Rosuvastatin
Salmeterol
Saquinavir
Sargramostin
Scopolamine
Secobarbital
Secretin
Selegiline
Sermorelin
Sertraline
Siberian ginseng
Sibutramine
Sildenafil
Simvastatin
Sirolimus
Smallpox vaccine
Sodium oxybate
Solifenacin
Somatropin
Sotalol

Sparfloxacin
Spironolactone
Stanozolol
Stavudine
Streptokinase
Streptomycin
Succimer
Sucralfate
Sulfadiazine
Sulfamethoxazole
Sulfasalazine
Sulfisoxazole
Sulfites
Sulindac
Sumatriptan
Tacrine
Tacrolimus
Tadalafil
Tamoxifen
Tamsulosin
Tegaserod
Telithromycin
Telmisartan
Temazepam
Temozolomide
Tenecteplase
Tenofovir
Terazosin
Terbinafine
Terbutaline
Terconazole
Teriparatide
Testosterone
Tetracycline
Thalidomide
Theophylline
Thiabendazole
Thioguanine
Thiopental
Thioridazine
Thiotepa
Thiothixene
Tiagabine
Ticlopidine

Timolol
Tinidazole
Tizanidine
Tinzaparin
Tiotropium
Tirofiban
Tobramycin
Tocainide
Tolazamide
Tolbutamide
Tolcapone
Tolmetin
Tolterodine
Topiramate
Topotecan
Toremifene
Torsemide
Tositumomab & iodine131
Tramadol
Trandolapril
Tranylcypromine
Trastuzumab
Travoprost
Trazodone
Treprostinil
Tretinoin
Triamterene
Triazolam
Trifluoperazine
Trimeprazine
Trimethadione
Trimethobenzamide
Trimethoprim
Trimetrexate
Trimipramine
Trioxsalen
Tripelennamine
Triprolidine
Triptorelin
Trovafloxacin
Turmeric
Unoprostone
Valacyclovir
Valdecoxib

Valganciclovir
Valproic acid
Valsartan
Vardenafil
Vasopressin
Venlafaxine
Verapamil
Vigabatrin
Vinblastine
Vincristine
Voriconazole
Warfarin
Zafirlukast
Zalcitabine
Zaleplon
Zanamivir
Zidovudine
Zileuton
Ziprasidone
Zoledronic acid
Zolmitriptan
Zolpidem
Zonisamide

HICCUPS
Amifostine
Aprepitant
Bretylium
Carisoprodol
Cevimeline
Ciprofloxacin
Cisplatin
Citalopram
Corticosteroids
Ethosuximide
Famotidine
Floxuridine
Fomepizole
Frovatriptan
Interferon beta-1A
Levodopa
Metaxalone
Methocarbamol
Methsuximide

Nicotine (>10%)
Nizatidine
Ondansetron
Oxaliplatin
Oxycodone
Palonosetron
Paramethadione
Pentazocine
Pergolide
Propoxyphene
Ranitidine

Mefloquine
Nafarelin (>10%)
Naproxen
Piroxicam
Progestins
Raloxifene (>10%)
Rasburicase
Rizatriptan
Ropinirole
Thiopental
Zolmitriptan (>10%)

HOT FLASHES

Cabergoline
Capecitabine
Celecoxib
Cetirizine
Cevimeline
Citalopram
Clomiphene (>10%)
Dihydroergotamine
Donepezil
Doxazosin
Duloxetine
Epirubicin (5–39%)
Etodolac
Exemestane (13%)
Flumazenil
Flurbiprofen
Frovatriptan
Fulvestrant (19–24%)
Goserelin (62–96%)
Granisetron
Ibuprofen
Indomethacin
Interferon beta-1B
Ketoprofen
Lamotrigine
Letrozole (5–19%)
Leuprolide
Levodopa
Meclofenamate
Medroxyprogesterone
Mefenamic acid

HYPERESTHESIA

Acebutolol
Acitretin (10–25%)
Abciximab
Acebutolol
Acitretin
Almotriptan
Alprostadil (<1%)
Amlodipine
Amprenavir
Arbutamine
Aripiprazole
Azelastine
Balsalazide
Basiliximab
Bexarotene
Bisoprolol
Bleomycin
Botulinum toxin (a & b)
Bupropion
Carvedilol
Celecoxib
Cetirizine
Cevimeline
Cilostazol
Citalopram
Clonidine
Clopidogrel
Cyanocobalamin
Cyclosporine
Delavirdine
Dipyridamole

Doxazosin
Doxycycline
Efavirenz
Eletriptan
Ertapenem
Esomeprazole
Exemestane
Flecainide
Flumazenil
Fluoxetine
Formoterol
Foscarnet
Fosphenytoin
Frovatriptan
Ganciclovir
Gatifloxacin
Gemfibrozil
Glatiramer
Glipizide
Grepafloxacin
Hepatitis B vaccine
Indinavir
Interferon alfa-2A
Interferon beta-1A
Interferon beta-1B
Isosorbide mononitrate
Labetalol
Lamotrigine
Levalbuterol
Levobupivacaine
Levofloxacin
Lomefloxacin
Loratadine
Losartan
Mephenytoin
Methysergide
Metoprolol
Midodrine
Minocycline
Mirtazapine
Moricizine
Morphine
Moxifloxacin
Myrrh

Nadolol
Naratriptan
Nefazodone
Nisoldipine
Norfloxacin
Octreotide
Ofloxacin
Olanzapine
Oxaliplatin
Oxcarbazepine
Oxytetracycline
Pantoprazole
Penbutolol
Phenindamine
Phenytoin
Pindolol
Pipecuronium
Pramipexole
Propranolol
Rapacuronium
Riluzole
Rimantadine
Risperidone
Ritonavir
Rituximab
Rivastigmine
Rizatriptan
Rofecoxib
Ropinirole
Saquinavir
Sertraline
Sildenafil
Sirolimus
Somatropin
Sparfloxacin
Sumatriptan
Tacrolimus
Tadalafil
Telmisartan
Thalidomide
Tolcapone
Topiramate
Trandolapril
Trastuzumab

Valdecoxib
Valproic acid
Venlafaxine
Verteporfin
Vinorelbine
Voriconazole
Zaleplon
Ziprasidone (<1%)
Zolmitriptan (<1%)
Zolpidem (<1%)
Zonisamide (<1%)

HYPERREFLEXIA
Almotriptan
Aripiprazole
Frovatriptan
Phenelzine
Zidovudine
Ziprasidone

HYPERTONIA
Aripiprazole
Baclofen
Balsalazide
Benazepril
Bicalutamide
Brinzolamide
Cefaclor
Celecoxib
Cevimeline
Citalopram
Cyclobenzaprine
Dicyclomine
Dipyridamole
Doxazosin
Esomeprazole
Fluvoxamine
Gatifloxacin
Glatirame (22%)
Glycopyrrolate
Interferon beta-1A
Interferon beta-1B
Levofloxacin
Lomefloxacin

Mesalamine
Mesna
Modafinil
Moxifloxacin
Mycophenolate
Nefazodone
Norfloxacin
Ofloxacin
Olanzapine
Pantoprazole
Peginterferon alfa-2B
Pramipexole
Propofol
Rituximab
Zalcitabine

HYPESTHESIA
Acebutolol
Acitretin (<1%)
Alosetron
Alprostadil (<1%)
Amprenavir
Atazanavir
Azacitidine
Basiliximab
Bexarotene
Carvedilol
Vardenafil
Celecoxib
Cetirizine
Citalopram
Duloxetine
Flecainide
Foscarnet
Frovatriptan
Gemifloxacin
Hepatitis B vaccine
Levalbuterol
Losartan
Mephenytoin
Montelukast
Phenytoin
Risperidone
Rituximab

Ropinirole
Zaleplon

HYPOKINESIA

Carvedilol
Citalopram
Entacapone
Galantamine
Memantine
Zalcitabine

IMPOTENCE

Acebutolol
Amoxapine
Aripiprazole
Atomoxetine
Baclofen
Basiliximab
Benazepril
Bepridil
Captopril
Carbamazepine
Carvedilol
Cevimeline
Chlorothiazide
Chlorpromazine
Citalopram
Clofibrate
Clonidine
Disulfiram
Doxazosin
Dutasteride
Enalapril
Escitalopram
Esomeprazole
Ethionamide
Felodipine
Finasteride
Flecainide
Flutamide
Fluvastatin
Fluvoxamine
Fosphenytoin
Gabapentin

Gemfibrozil
Glycopyrrolate
Goserelin
Hydralazine
Hyoscyamine
Imipramine
Indapamide
Interferon alfa-2A
Interferon beta-1B
Isosorbide mononitrate
Isradipine
Itraconazole
Ketoconazole
Labetalol
Lamotrigine
Leuprolide
Lisinopril
Losartan
Lovastatin
Mepenzolate
Mesoridazine
Methantheline
Methazolamide
Methyltestosterone
Metolazone
Metoprolol
Mexiletine
Misoprostol
Mitoxantrone
Moexipril
Mycophenolate
Nabumetone
Nadolol
Naltrexone
Nefazodone
Nisoldipine
Nortriptyline
Oxaprozin
Oxybutynin
Paroxetine
Penbutolol
Perindopril
Perphenazine
Phentermine

Pindolol
Pramipexole
Pravastatin
Primidone
Prochlorperazine
Promazine
Promethazine
Propantheline
Propranolol
Protriptyline
Quinapril
Quinethazone
Ramipril
Reserpine
Ropinirole
Venlafaxine
Ziprasidone

JOINT PAIN
Anthrax vaccine
Apomorphine
Ascorbic acid
Bortezomib
Calcitonin
Cefaclor
Cephradine
Ciprofloxacin
Clopidogrel
Collagen
Cyclophosphamide
Cytarabine
Daclizumab
Danazol
Daptomycin
Darbepoetin alfa
Daunorubicin
Denileukin
Dicloxacillin
Dicumarol
Dimenhydrinate
Dofetilide
Doxorubicin
Duloxetine
Efavirenz

Emtricitabine
Epirubicin
Eplerenone
Eprosartan
Escitalopram
Esomeprazole
Etanercept
Ethacrynic acid
Ethotoin
Exemestane
Ezetimibe
Fluorides
Fondaparinux
Fosamprenavir
Fosinopril
Fosphenytoin
Furazolidone
Furosemide
Gabapentin
Gadodiamide
Gefitinib
Glatiramer
Goserelin
Hydralazine
Hydrochlorothiazide
Hydroflumethiazide
Hydroxyurea
Ibandronate
Idarubicin
Imatinib (27%)
Immune globulin IV
Interferon alfa-2A
Interferon beta-1A
Isotretinoin
Itraconazole
Ivermectin
Lansoprazole
Latanoprost
Levamisole
Mechlorethamine
Memantine
Mephenytoin
Mercaptopurine
Mesalamine

Methicillin
Methyclothiazide
Methyldopa
Mezlocillin
Montelukast
Nafcillin
Nalidixic acid
Naltrexone
Naratriptan
Natalizumab
Nateglinide
Nefazodone
Niacin
Nicotine
Nitrofurantoin
Olmesartan
Omalizumab
Omeprazole
Oxacillin
Oxcarbazepine
Paclitaxel
Palifermin
Palonosetron
Pamidronate
Paramethadione
Paroxetine
Pegfilgrastim
Pegvisomant
Pemetrexed
Penicillins
Pentostatin
Perindopril
Phenytoin
Pilocarpine
Pimecrolimus
Piperacillin
Polythiazide
Potassium iodide
Pramipexole
Praziquantel
Probenecid
Procarbazine
Propantheline
Quinidine

Quinupristin/Dalfopristin
Raloxifene
Repaglinide
Ribavirin
Rifapentine
Risedronate
Ritonavir
Ropinirole
Sargramostin
Secobarbital
Stavudine
Streptokinase
Sulfadiazine
Sulfadoxine
Sulfamethoxazole
Sulfasalazine
Sulfinpyrazone
Tacrolimus
Tadalafil
Tegaserod
Telithromycin
Thiabendazole
Thioguanine
Tinidazole
Tinzaparin
Tiopronin
Tizanidine
Trientine
Trimethadione
Trimethoprim
Unoprostone
Valsartan
Vigabatrin
Zafirlukast
Zanamivir
Zidovudine

LEG PAIN
Atenolol
Basiliximab
Botulinum toxin (a & b)
Carteolol
Celecoxib
Cetirizine

Citalopram
Clofarabine (29%)
Cyclosporine
Diethylstilbestrol
Enflurane
Enoxaparin
Ertapenem
Escitalopram
Estramustine
Estrogens
Halothane
Isoflurane
Ketamine
Labetalol
Losartan
Mesalamine
Mesna
Methohexital
Methoxyflurane
Metoprolol
Nadolol
Omalizumab
Penbutolol
Pindolol
Propofol
Propranolol
Sargramostin
Sirolimus
Tadalafil
Tegaserod
Thiopental
Toremifene
Triptorelin

MIGRAINE
Albuterol
Allopurinol
Amlodipine
Aripiprazole
Botulinum toxin (a & b)
Calcitonin
Capecitabine
Carvedilol
Celecoxib

Cetirizine
Cevimeline
Chlorotrianisene
Ciprofloxacin
Citalopram
Clomipramine
Cyclosporine
Dofetilide
Epoetin alfa
Eprosartan
Esomeprazole
Estrogens
Felbamate
Fenofibrate
Gatifloxacin
Glatiramer
Goserelin
Hepatitis B vaccine
Interferon beta-1A
Isoetharine
Lamotrigine
Levalbuterol
Levofloxacin
Lomefloxacin
Medroxyprogesterone
Moxifloxacin
Niacin
Nisoldipine
Norfloxacin
Ofloxacin
Oxcarbazepine
Pantoprazole
Paroxetine
Perindopril
Phenindamine
Progestins
Raloxifene
Ritonavir
Rivastigmine
Tartrazine
Tizanidine
Zalcitabine

MULTIPLE SCLEROSIS
Adalimumab (5%)
Hepatitis B vaccine

MYALGIA
Aprepitant
Baclofen
Bumetanide
Cefaclor
Cevimeline
Cidofovir
Citalopram
Collagen
Daclizumab
Dihydrotachysterol
Dofetilide
Doxazosin
Doxercalciferol
Efavirenz
Emtricitabine
Entacapone
Ephedrine
Epinephrine
Eplerenone
Ergocalciferol
Escitalopram
Estrogens
Ethacrynic acid
Ethosuximide
Etodolac
Ezetimibe
Fenofibrate
Fluoxetine
Flurbiprofen
Fondaparinux
Fosamprenavir
Fosphenytoin
Frovatriptan
Gabapentin
Galantamine
Gefitinib
Gemcitabine
Gemfibrozil
Gemifloxacin

Gemtuzumab
Glucagon
Goserelin
Guanadrel
Hydralazine
Hydrochlorothiazide
Hydroflumethiazide
Ibandronate
Ibritumomab
Ibuprofen
Imatinib (11–46%)
Imiquimod
Immune globulin IV
Indapamide
Indomethacin
Infliximab
Interferon beta-1B
Irbesartan
Itraconazole
Ivermectin
Ketoconazole
Ketoprofen
Lamivudine (>10%)
Lamotrigine
Lansoprazole
Latanoprost
Letrozole (>10%)
Levalbuterol
Levamisole
Meclofenamate
Mefenamic acid
Memantine
Mephenytoin
Metformin
Methsuximide
Methyclothiazide
Mirtazapine
Nafarelin
Nalidixic acid
Naproxen
Naratriptan
Natalizumab
Nateglinide
Nicotine

Nitrofurantoin
Olmesartan
Omalizumab
Omeprazole
Oxcarbazepine
Paclitaxel
Palivizumab
Palonosetron
Pamidronate
Pantoprazole
Paramethadione
Paroxetine
Peginterferon alfa-2B
Pegvisomant
Pemetrexed
Penicillins
Pergolide
Phenytoin
Pilocarpine
Pimecrolimus
Pindolol (10%)
Piroxicam
Polythiazide
Pramipexole
Procarbazine
Quinidine
Quinupristin/Dalfopristin
Raloxifene
Reteplase
Ribavirin
Rifabutin
Rifampin
Riluzole
Rosuvastatin
Salmeterol
Sargramostin
Secobarbital
Simvastatin
Sodium oxybate
Somatropin
Sotalol
Spironolactone
Stavudine
Streptokinase

Sulfadoxine
Sulfasalazine
Sumatriptan
Tacrine
Tacrolimus
Tadalafil
Telithromycin
Temazepam
Thiabendazole
Tiagabine
Tinidazole
Tinzaparin
Tiopronin
Tiotropium
Tizanidine
Topotecan
Torsemide
Trandolapril
Travoprost
Trazodone
Triazolam
Trimeprazine
Trimetrexate
Unoprostone
Valdecoxib
Vigabatrin
Voriconazole
Zafirlukast
Zalcitabine
Zaleplon
Zidovudine
Ziprasidone
Zoledronic acid
Zolpidem (7%)
Zonisamide

MYASTHENIA

Adalimumab
Betaxolol
Bexarotene
Bicalutamide
Botulinum toxin (a & b)
Captopril
Carmustine

Cefoxitin (exacerbation)
Gatifloxacin
Glatiramer
Interferon beta-1B (46%)
Levobetaxolol
Levobunolol
Levofloxacin
Lithium
Lomefloxacin
Metipranolol
Metolazone
Moxifloxacin
Mycophenolate
Nelfinavir
Norfloxacin
Ofloxacin
Paroxetine
Penicillamine
Pilocarpine
Pramipexole
Quinupristin/Dalfopristin
Risedronate
Rosuvastatin
Telithromycin
Thiopental

NECK PAIN
Anastrozole
Botulinum toxin (a & b) (11%)
Carmustine
Cefaclor
Chlorpromazine
Ciprofloxacin
Hepatitis B vaccine
Lamotrigine
Modafinil
Pantoprazole
Rizatriptan
Rosuvastatin
Streptokinase
Temazepam
Teriparatide
Tizanidine
Tranylcypromine

Triazolam
Zalcitabine

NEURALGIA
Calcitonin
Celecoxib
Cilostazol
Citalopram
Clofazimine
Clopidogrel
Efavirenz
Felodipine
Fenofibrate
Glatiramer
Isradipine
Oxcarbazepine
Rabeprazole
Zalcitabine

NEURITIS
Allopurinol (<1%)
Amlodipine
Cytarabine
Emtricitabine
Eprosartan
Ethambutol
Ethionamide
Infliximab
Pergolide
Propylthiouracil
Rituximab
Zalcitabine

NEUROLEPTIC MALIGNANT SYNDROME
Amitriptyline
Amoxapine
Chlorpromazine
Citalopram
Clozapine
Donepezil
Droperidol
Fluoxetine
Haloperidol

Loxapine
Mesoridazine
Methylphenidate
Metoclopramide
Molindone
Olanzapine
Paroxetine
Pergolide
Perphenazine
Prochlorperazine
Promazine
Promethazine
Risperidone

NEUROPATHY
Almotriptan
Aripiprazole
Basiliximab
Bexarotene
Bicalutamide
Carboplatin
Celecoxib
Cevimeline
Delavirdine
Disopyramide
Disulfiram
Docetaxel
Efavirenz
Emtricitabine
Enfuvirtide
Etodolac
Etoposide
Flecainide
Flucytosine
Fluvastatin
Fluvoxamine
Foscarnet
Ganciclovir
Gemifloxacin
Gemtuzumab
Gold
Heparin
Hydroxyurea
Ibuprofen

Imipramine
Indomethacin
Infliximab
Interferon alfa-2A
Lamivudine (>10%)
Levofloxacin
Linezolid
Lisinopril
Lomefloxacin
Losartan
Lovastatin
Meclofenamate
Methotrexate
Misoprostol
Moexipril
Monosodium glutamate
Moxifloxacin
Mycophenolate
Naproxen
Norfloxacin
Nortriptyline
Ofloxacin
Oxaliplatin (48%)
Paclitaxel
Pemetrexed (17–29%)
Penicillamine
Perindopril
Phenytoin
Piroxicam
Pravastatin
Procainamide
Procarbazine (>10%)
Propantheline
Protriptyline
Quinapril
Quinethazone
Quinupristin/Dalfopristin
Rabeprazole
Ramipril
Ritonavir
Rituximab
Rivastigmine
Rizatriptan

NEUROTOXICITY

Altretamine (21%)
Amikacin
Cladribine
Kanamycin
Lomustine
Neomycin
Nimodipine
Streptomycin

PAIN

Abarelix (31%)
Acamprosate (5%)
Acebutolol
Acitretin (10%)
Abarelix
Acamprosate
Adalimumab (<5%)
Adefovir
Agalsidase (21%)
Albendazol
Albuterol
Aldesleukin (>10%)
Alefacept
Alemtuzumab (24%)
Alendronate
Alfuzosin (1–2%)
Alitretinoin (<34%)
Allopurinol IV
Alosetron
Alprostadil (2–10%)
Aminolevulinic acid
Amphotericin B
Anagrelide
Anastrozole
Arbutamine
Argatroban
Arsenic
Atazanavir
Azacitidine
Balsalazide
Basiliximab
Bepridil
Bevacizumab

Bexarotene
Bicalutamide
Bismuth
Bivalirudin (15%)
Bortezomib
Botulinum toxin (a & b) (6–13%)
Cabergoline
Capecitabine (12%)
Capreomycin
Capsicum
Carboplatin
Carmustine (13%)
Carvedilol
Cascara
Caspofungin
Cefditoren
Ceftizoxime
Ceftriaxone
Celecoxib
Cetirizine
Cetuximab (17%)
Cevimeline
Chlortetracycline
Cidofovir (25%)
Ciprofloxacin
Cladribine
Clofarabine
Colchicine
Corticosteroids
Cyanocobalamin
Daclizumab
Dalteparin
Danaparoid
Dantrolene
Daptomycin
Denileukin (48%)
Dexmedetomidine
Dextroamphetamine
Diclofenac (topical: 15–26%)
Dihydroergotamine
Dinoprostone
Docetaxel
Dolasetron
Donepezil

Doxazosin
Doxorubicin
Efalizumab (10%)
Efavirenz
Enfuvirtide
Enoxaparin
Epinastine
Epoetin alfa
Ertapenem
Etanercept
Exemestane (13%)
Felbamate
Fenofibrate
Fexofenadine
Fondaparinux
Frovatriptan
Fulvestrant
Gadodiamide
Gemcitabine (40%)
Gemtuzumab (25%)
Glatiramer (28%)
Goserelin (8–17%)
Granisetron
Heparin
Hepatitis b vaccine
Ibritumomab (13%)
Imiquimod
Infliximab
Interferon beta-1A (20%)
Interferon beta-1B (51%)
Isoetharine
Lamotrigine
Laronidase
Levalbuterol
Levetiracetam
Letrozole (5%)
Leuprolide
Levobupivacaine (7–18%)
Mafenide
Medroxyprogesterone
Memantine
Mesalamine (14%)
Methadone
Methamphetamine

Midodrine
Morphine
Mupirocin
Mycophenolate (31–76%)
Nafcillin
Nalbuphine
Nelfinavir
Olmesartan
Omalizumab
Oxaliplatin (14%)
Paclitaxel (17%)
Palifermin (16%)
Pantoprazole
Peginterferon alfa-2B (12%)
Pegvisomant (4–14%)
Pemetrexed
Pentostatin
Perflutren
Pergolide
Phenytoin
Pilocarpine
Pimecrolimus
Piperacillin
Quetiapine
Quinupristin/Dalfopristin
Rabeprazole
Rasburicase
Rifapentine
Rifaximin
Riluzole
Rituximab (12%)
Rosuvastatin
Sermorelin
Sodium oxybate
Somatropin
Streptozocin
Succimer
Tacrolimus
Tadalafil
Tegaserod
Telithromycin
Tenofovir
Terazosin
Teriparatide

Thiotepa
Tiagabine
Tinidazole
Tinzaparin
Tositumomab & iodine 131
Trastuzumab
Travoprost
Treprostinil
Tretinoin
Troleandomycin
Trovafloxacin
Vardenafil
Vasopressin
Verteporfin
Vidarabine
Voriconazole
Zanamivir
Zoledronic acid

PARALYSIS

Alemtuzumab
Allopurinol IV
Balsalazide
Cetirizine
Cevimeline
Dalteparin
Danaparoid
Delavirdine
Dofetilide
Enoxaparin
Fluvoxamine
Glatiramer
Ibritumomab
Lamotrigine
Lovastatin
Methotrexate
Peginterferon alfa-2B
Quinupristin/Dalfopristin
Rasburicase
Sirolimus
Streptomycin
Tinzaparin
Zalcitabine

PARESTHESIAS

Acamprosate (2%)
Acetazolamide
Acetohexamide
Acitretin (10–25%)
Acyclovir (<1%)
Abacavir
Acamprosate
Acetazolamide
Acetohexamide
Acitretin
Acyclovir
Adalimumab (5%)
Adenosine (1%)
Agalsidase (14%)
Alitretinoin (3–22%)
Allopurinol (<1%)
Almotriptan (1%)
Alprazolam (2.4%)
Altretamine
Amantadine
Amikacin (<1%)
Amiloride
Amiodarone
Amitriptyline
Amlodipine
Amoxapine
Amphotericin B
Amprenavir
Anagrelide
Anastrozole
Anthrax vaccine
Apraclonidine
Arbutamine
Aripiprazole
Arsenic
Aspirin
Atomoxetine
Atorvastatin
Azatadine
Azithromycin
Aztreonam
Baclofen
Basiliximab

Benactyzine
Benazepril
Bendroflumethiazide
Benzthiazide
Benztropine
Bepridil
Betaxolol
Bicalutamide
Biperiden
Bisoprolol
Bleomycin
Bortezomib (23%)
Bromocriptine
Brompheniramine
Bupropion
Buspirone
Butorphanol
Cabergoline
Caffeine
Calcitonin
Candesartan
Capecitabine (12%)
Captopril
Carbamazepine
Carisoprodol
Carteolol
Carvedilol
Caspofungin
Cefaclor
Cefamandole
Cefotaxime
Cefpodoxime
Cefprozil
Ceftazidime
Ceftibuten
Ceftazidime
Ceftizoxime
Celecoxib
Cephapirin
Cetirizine
Cevimeline
Chloramphenicol
Chlordiazepoxide
Chlorothiazide

Chlorpheniramine
Chlorpropamide
Chlorthalidone
Cholestyramine
Cholestyramine
Cidofovir (> 10%)
Cilostazol
Cinoxacin
Ciprofloxacin
Citalopram
Clemastine
Clomipramine
Clonazepam
Clopidogrel
Clorazepate
Clonazepam
Clopidogrel
Cocaine
Codeine
Colchicine
Corticosteroids
Cromolyn
Cyanocobalamin
Cyclamate
Cyclobenzaprine
Cycloserine
Cyclosporine
Cyclothiazide
Cyproheptadine
Cytarabine
Dacarbazine
Dalteparin
Danaparoid
Danazol
Dapsone
Daptomycin
Delavirdine
Demeclocycline
Denileukin (13%)
Desipramine
Dexchlorpheniramine
Diazepam
Diazoxide
Diclofenac (topical: 8–20%)

Dicumarol
Didanosine
Diethylpropion
Diflunisal
Dihydroergotamine (>10%)
Diltiazem
Dimenhydrinate
Dimercaprol
Dinoprostone
Diphenhydramine
Diphenoxylate
Dipyridamole
Dirithromycin
Disopyramide
Disulfiram
Dobutamine
Docetaxel
Dofetilide
Dolasetron
Donepezil
Dorzolamide
Doxapram
Doxazosin
Doxepin
Doxorubicin
Doxycycline
Dronabinol
Duloxetine
Echinacea
Efavirenz
Eflornithine
Eletriptan
Emtricitabine
Enalapril
Enfuvirtide
Enoxacin
Enoxaparin
Eplerenone
Epoetin alfa (11%)
Eprosartan
Ertapenem
Escitalopram
Esmolol
Esomeprazole

Estazolam
Estrogens
Ethacrynic acid
Ethambutol
Ethchlorvynol
Ethionamide
Ethotoin
Etidronate
Etodolac
Etoposide
Exemestane
Famciclovir
Famotidine
Felbamate
Felodipine
Fenofibrate
Fentanyl
Flecainide
Floxuridine
Fluconazole
Flucytosine
Fludarabine (>10%)
Flumazenil
Fluorouracil
Fluoxetine
Fluoxymesterone
Flurazepam
Flurbiprofen
Flutamide
Fluvastatin
Fluvoxamine
Fondaparinux
Fosamprenavir
Foscarnet
Fosfomycin
Fosinopril
Fosphenytoin
Frovatriptan
Fulvestrant
Furosemide
Gabapentin
Gadodiamide
Galantamine
Ganciclovir

Gatifloxacin
Gefitinib
Gemcitabine (10%)
Gemfibrozil
Gemifloxacin
Gemtuzumab
Gentamicin
Glatiramer
Glipizide
Glyburide
Gold
Goserelin
Grepafloxacin
Griseofulvin
Guanadrel (25%)
Guanethidine
Guanfacine
Hepatitis B vaccine
Hydralazine
Hydrochlorothiazide
Hydrocodone
Hydroflumethiazide
Hydromorphone
Hydroxyzine
Ibandronate
Ibuprofen
Idarubicin
Imatinib (<10%)
Imipenem/Cilastatin
Imipramine
Indapamide
Indinavir
Indomethacin
Infliximab
Insulin
Interferon alfa-2A
Interferon beta-1A
Interferon beta-1B
Ipratropium
Irbesartan
Irinotecan
Isoniazid
Isotretinoin
Isradipine

Itraconazole
Kanamycin (<1%)
Ketoconazole
Ketoprofen
Ketorolac
Labetalol
Lamivudine (>10%)
Lamotrigine
Lansoprazole
Laronidase (14%)
Leflunomide
Leuprolide
Levalbuterol
Levamisole
Levetiracetam
Levobupivacaine
Levodopa
Levofloxacin
Lidocaine
Lindane
Lisinopril
Lomefloxacin
Loratadine
Lorazepam
Losartan
Lovastatin
Loxapine
Mazindol
MDMA
Mecamylamine
Mechlorethamine
Meclizine
Meclofenamate
Medroxyprogesterone
Mefenamic acid
Mefloquine
Meloxicam
Meperidine
Mephenytoin
Meprobamate
Mesalamine
Mesoridazine
Methadone
Methazolamide

Methimazole
Methyclothiazide
Methyldopa
Methyltestosterone
Methysergide
Metoclopramide
Metolazone
Metoprolol
Metronidazole
Mexiletine
Midazolam
Midodrine (18%)
Miglustat
Minocycline
Minoxidil
Mirtazapine
Mitomycin
Modafinil
Moexipril
Monosodium glutamate
Montelukast
Moricizine
Morphine
Moxifloxacin
Mycophenolate (21%)
Nabumetone
Nadolol
Nafarelin
Nalbuphine
Nalidixic acid
Naproxen
Naratriptan
Nebivolol
Nefazodone
Nelfinavir
Neomycin
Nesiritide
Nevirapine
Niacin
Niacinamide (<10%)
Nicardipine
Nicotine
Nifedipine
Nisoldipine

Nitrofurantoin
Nizatidine
Norfloxacin
Nortriptyline
Octreotide
Ofloxacin
Olmesartan
Omalizumab
Omeprazole
Ondansetron
Orphenadrine
Oxaliplatin
Oxaprozin
Oxazepam
Oxybutynin
Oxycodone
Oxytetracycline
Paclitaxel (>10%)
Palifermin
Palonosetron
Pantoprazole
Paramethadione
Paroxetine
Peginterferon alfa-2B
Pegvisomant
Pemetrexed
Penbutolol
Pentagastrin
Pentazocine
Pentostatin
Pentoxifylline
Perflutren
Pergolide
Perindopril
Phenindamine
Phenylephrine
Phenytoin
Pindolol
Pirbuterol
Piroxicam
Polythiazide
Potassium iodide
Pramipexole
Pravastatin

Prazepam
Prazosin
Procarbazine (>10%)
Promethazine
Propafenone
Propofol
Propoxyphene
Propranolol
Propylthiouracil
Protriptyline
Pyridoxine
Pyrilamine
Quazepam
Quetiapine
Quinapril
Quinethazone
Quinine
Quinupristin/dalfopristin
Rabeprazole
Ramipril
Ranitidine
Rasburicase
Repaglinide
Reserpine
Reteplase
Rifabutin
Riluzole
Risedronate
Risperidone
Ritonavir
Rituximab
Rivastigmine
Rizatriptan
Rofecoxib
Ropinirole
Rosuvastatin
Salmeterol
Saquinavir
Secretin
Selegiline
Selenium
Sertraline
Sibutramine
Sildenafil

Simvastatin
Sirolimus
Sodium oxybate
Somatropin
Sotalol
Sparfloxacin
Spironolactone
St John's wort
Stavudine
Streptokinase
Streptomycin
Succimer
Sulindac
Sumatriptan
Tacrine
Tacrolimus
Tadalafil
Tartrazine
Telithromycin
Telmisartan
Temazepam
Temozolomide
Tenofovir
Terazosin
Terfenadine
Teriparatide
Testosterone
Tetracycline
Thalidomide
Thiabendazole
Thiamine
Thioridazine
Thiothixene
Tiagabine
Timolol
Tinidazole
Tinzaparin
Tiotropium
Tizanidine
Tobramycin
Tocainide
Tolazamide
Tolbutamide
Tolcapone

Tolterodine
Topiramate
Topotecan
Tramadol
Trandolapril
Tranylcypromine
Trastuzumab
Trazodone
Tretinoin
Triamterene
Triazolam
Trichlormethiazide
Trihexyphenidyl
Trimeprazine
Trimethadione
Trimipramine
Tripelennamine
Triprolidine
Trovafloxacin
Trazodone
Trimethadione
Trimetrexate
Trimipramine
Unoprostone
Valacyclovir
Valdecoxib
Valganciclovir
Valproic acid
Valsartan
Vancomycin
Vardenafil
Venlafaxine
Verapamil
Verteporfin
Vigabatrin
Vinblastine
Vincristine
Vinorelbine
Voriconazole
Zalcitabine
Zaleplon
Zidovudine (1–10%)
Zileuton
Ziprasidone (<1%)

Zoledronic acid
Zolmitriptan (11%)
Zolpidem (<1%)
Zonisamide (4%)

PARKINSONISM
Amitriptyline
Apomorphine
Asparaginase
Bupropion
Carboplatin
Citalopram
Cyclosporine
Desipramine
Diltiazem
Donepezil
Doxepin
Entacapone (17%)
Flucytosine
Fluphenazine
Imipramine
Infliximab
Interferon alfa-2A
Kava
Lamotrigine
Lithium
Loxapine
Maprotiline
MDMA
Methyldopa
Metoclopramide
Nabumetone
Nortriptyline
Olanzapine
Oxaprozin
Pemoline
Phenelzine
Protriptyline
Reserpine
Risperidone
Ritonavir

PAROSMIA
Amikacin

Amiodarone
Apraclonidine
Balsalazide
Betaxolol
Calcitonin
Cetirizine
Cevimeline
Ciprofloxacin
Cocaine (>10%)
Doxazosin
Doxycycline
Dronabinol
Efavirenz
Enalapril
Eletriptan
Esomeprazole
Fluoxetine
Flurbiprofen
Fluvoxamine
Fomepizole
Gatifloxacin
Interferon alfa-2A
Interferon beta-1A
Interferon beta-1B
Isotretinoin
Kanamycin
Levamisole
Levobetaxolol
Levobunolol
Levofloxacin
Lomefloxacin
Methazolamide
Metipranolol
Metolazone
Minocycline
Minoxidil
Mirtazapine
Moxifloxacin
Neomycin
Nifedipine
Norfloxacin
Ofloxacin
Oxytetracycline
Paroxetine

Pentamidine
Pravastatin
Propantheline
Rimantadine
Ritonavir
Zaleplon
Zolmitriptan (<1%)
Zonisamide (<1%)

PENILE PAIN
Alprostadil (37%)
Ginseng
Sildenafil

PERIPHERAL NEUROPATHY
Allopurinol (<1%)
Bortezomib (37%)
Capecitabine (10%)
Carbamazepine
Chlorambucil
Cisplatin (>10%)
Disulfiram
Streptomycin
Thalidomide
Zalcitabine

PEYRONIE'S DISEASE
Atenolol
Betaxolol
Bisoprolol
Carteolol
Labetalol
Levobetaxolol
Levobunolol
Metipranolol
Metolazone
Metoprolol
Nadolol
Penbutolol
Phenytoin
Pindolol
Propranolol
Ropinirole

PRIAPISM
  Androstenedione
  Anisindione
  Aripiprazole
  Bupropion
  Chlorpromazine
  Citalopram
  Clozapine
  Cocaine
  Codeine
  Dicumarol
  Doxazosin
  Droperidol
  Fluoxetine
  Fluoxymesterone (>10%)
  Fluphenazine
  Fluvoxamine
  Gabapentin
  Glatiramer
  Guanfacine
  Haloperidol
  Hydrocodone
  Hydroxyzine
  Labetalol
  Levodopa
  Loxapine
  MDMA
  Meperidine
  Mesoridazine
  Methadone
  Methyltestosterone (>10%)
  Metoprolol
  Molindone
  Morphine
  Nadolol
  Nalbuphine
  Nefazodone
  Olanzapine
  Oxcarbazepine
  Oxycodone
  Papaverine (11%)
  Paroxetine
  Penbutolol
  Pentazocine

  Pergolide
  Perphenazine
  Phenelzine
  Phenoxybenzamine
  Pindolol
  Prazosin
  Prochlorperazine
  Promazine
  Promethazine
  Propoxyphene
  Propranolol
  Quetiapine
  Risperidone (<10%)
  Sildenafil
  Stanozolol
  Tadalafil
  Tamsulosin
  Terazosin
  Trazodone
  Vardenafil
  Ziprasidone

PSEUDOPARKINSONISM
  Chlorpromazine
  Droperidol
  Haloperidol
  Mesoridazine
  Molindone
  Perphenazine
  Prochlorperazine
  Promazine
  Promethazine
  Risperidone

PSEUDOTUMOR CEREBRI
  Acitretin (<1%)
  Acitretin
  Amiodarone
  Corticosteroids
  Cytarabine
  Demeclocycline
  Desmopressin
  Doxycycline
  Gentamicin

Isotretinoin
Kanamycin
Levothyroxine
Lindane
Liothyronine
Lithium
Mesalamine
Minocycline
Nalidixic acid
Neomycin
Nitrofurantoin
Oxytetracycline
Somatropin
Tetracycline
Tretinoin
Vitamin A

PTOSIS
Cetirizine
Citalopram

RIGORS
Acitretin (10–25%)
Agalsidase (52%)
Aldesleukin (>10%)
Alemtuzumab (86%)
Amifostine
Amlodipine
Amphotericin B
Arsenic
Atomoxetine
Azacitidine
Baclofen
Basiliximab
Bortezomib (12%)
Ceftibuten
Cetirizine
Cevimeline
Citalopram
Chlordiazepoxide
Chlorpromazine
Clofarabine
Clozapine
Daptomycin

Dipyridamole
Doxazosin
Duloxetine
Esmolol
Famciclovir
Foscarnet
Frovatriptan
Gadodiamide
Imatinib (8–11%)
Immune globulin IV
Interferon beta-1A (10%)
Loratadine
Mesoridazine
Misoprostol
Morphine
Natalizumab
Nefazodone
Olanzapine
Oxaliplatin
Peginterferon alfa-2B (23–45%)
Perphenazine
Phenindamine
Prochlorperazine
Promethazine
Rasburicase
Rituximab
Ziprasidone

SEIZURES
Acetazolamide
Acetylcysteine
Acyclovir (<1%)
Aldesleukin (<1%)
Alemtuzumab
Alendronate
Allopurinol IV
Alprostadil (1–10%)
Alteplase
Altretamine (1–10%)
Amantadine (<1%)
Aminocaproic acid
Aminophylline
Amoxapine
Amoxicillin

Amphotericin B
Ampicillin
Androstenedione
Anthrax vaccine
Aprotinin
Arsenic
Aspirin
Azithromycin
Aztreonam
Baclofen
Benzonatate
Bethanechol
Black cohosh
Bortezomib
Bromocriptine
Bupropion
Buspirone
Carbamazepine
Carbinoxamine
Carvedilol
Cefaclor
Cefazolin
Cefepime
Ceftazidime
Ceftizoxime
Ceftriaxone
Cefuroxime
Cetirizine
Cevimeline
Chlorambucil
Chloroquine
Chlorpromazine
Cidofovir
Cinacalcet
Ciprofloxacin
Cisplatin
Citalopram
Clarithromycin
Clomipramine
Clonazepam
Clozapine
Co-Trimoxazole
Cocaine
Codeine

Corticosteroids
Cyclobenzaprine
Cycloserine
Cyclosporine
Cyproheptadine
Cytarabine
Dantrolene
Daptomycin
Darbepoetin alfa
Deferoxamine
Desipramine
Desmopressin
Dicloxacillin
Dicyclomine
Didanosine
Diethylpropion
Diflunisal
Dihydroergotamine
Dimenhydrinate
Dimercaprol
Donepezil
Doxazosin
Doxepin
Doxorubicin
Dronabinol
Droperidol
Duloxetine
Edrophonium
Eflornithine
Eletriptan
Enflurane
Enoxaparin
Ephedrine
Epinephrine
Epoetin alfa
Ertapenem
Erythromycin
Escitalopram
Esmolol
Estrogens
Etanercept
Ethacrynic acid
Ethosuximide
Ethotoin

Etodolac
Famotidine
Fentanyl
Flecainide
Floxuridine
Fluconazole
Flumazenil
Fluoxetine
Fluphenazine
Flurazepam
Flurbiprofen
Fluvoxamine
Fomepizole
Fondaparinux
Foscarnet (>10%)
Fosphenytoin
Gabapentin
Gadodiamide
Galantamine
Ganciclovir
Gatifloxacin
Gemfibrozil
Gemifloxacin
Gemtuzumab
Gentamicin
Ginkgo biloba
Glatiramer
Glimepiride
Glipizide
Glyburide
Glycopyrrolate
Gold
Goldenseal
Guarana
Haloperidol
Hepatitis B vaccine
Heroin
Horse chestnut (seed)
Hydrochlorothiazide
Hydrocodone
Hydroflumethiazide
Hydroxychloroquine
Hydroxyurea
Hydroxyzine

Hyoscyamine
Ibandronate
Ibuprofen
Idarubicin
Imatinib
Imipramine
Immune globulin IV
Indomethacin
Infliximab
Insulin
Interferon alfa-2A
Interferon beta-1A
Interferon beta-1B
Irinotecan
Isocarboxazid
Isoniazid
Isosorbide dinitrate
Isosorbide mononitrate
Itraconazole
Kava
Ketoconazole
Ketoprofen
Ketorolac
Lamotrigine
Lansoprazole
Leucovorin
Leuprolide
Levalbuterol
Levamisole
Levetiracetam
Levobupivacaine
Levodopa
Levofloxacin
Levothyroxine
Lidocaine
Lindane
Liothyronine
Lithium
Lomefloxacin
Loracarbef
Loratadine
Loxapine
Maprotiline
Mazindol

Mebendazole
Mecamylamine
Meclofenamate
Medroxyprogesterone
Mefenamic acid
Mefloquine
Melatonin
Meloxicam
Mepenzolate
Meperidine
Mephenytoin
Mesoridazine
Methadone
Methantheline
Methazolamide
Methicillin
Methocarbamol
Methotrexate
Methsuximide
Methyclothiazide
Methysergide
Metoclopramide
Mexiletine
Mezlocillin
Midazolam
Misoprostol
Mitoxantrone
Molindone
Montelukast
Morphine
Moxifloxacin
Nabumetone
Nafcillin
Nalbuphine
Nalidixic acid
Naloxone
Naproxen
Naratriptan
Natalizumab
Nateglinide
Nitisinone
Nitroglycerin
Nizatidine
Norfloxacin

Nortriptyline
Octreotide
Ofloxacin
Olanzapine
Ondansetron
Oseltamivir
Oxacillin
Oxaprozin
Oxcarbazepine
Oxybutynin
Paclitaxel
Palonosetron
Pantoprazole
Paroxetine
Pemetrexed
Pemoline
Penicillins
Pentazocine
Pentostatin
Pentoxifylline
Pergolide
Perphenazine
Phendimetrazine
Phenindamine
Phentermine
Phenytoin
Physostigmine
Pimozide
Piperacillin
Piroxicam
Polythiazide
Procarbazine (>10%)
Prochlorperazine
Procyclidine
Promazine
Promethazine
Propantheline
Propoxyphene
Protriptyline
Pseudoephedrine
Pyridoxine
Pyrimethamine
Quinidine
Quinine

Quinupristin/Dalfopristin
Rabeprazole
Ramipril
Ranitidine
Rasburicase
Repaglinide
Reteplase
Riluzole
Risperidone
Ritonavir
Rivastigmine
Rosiglitazone
Rue
Secretin
Sertraline
Sibutramine
Sirolimus
Streptokinase
Sufentanil
Temozolomide
Theophylline
Thiabendazole
Thiopental
Thioridazine
Thiothixene
Ticarcillin
Tinidazole
Tizanidine
Topiramate
Tramadol
Trifluoperazin
Trimetrexate
Trimipramine
Trovafloxacin
Vasopressin
Vigabatrin
Voriconazole
Zalcitabine
Zanamivir
Zidovudine
Zoledronic acid
Zolpidem

SIALORRHEA
Acamprosate
Acitretin
Almotriptan
Alprazolam
Amiodarone
Amitriptyline
Amoxapine
Amoxicillin
Aprepitant
Aripiprazole
Betaxolol
Bethanechol
Bupropion
Buspirone
Carbachol
Cefpodoxime
Cetirizine
Cevimeline
Chlordiazepoxide
Cholestyramine
Citalopram
Clomipramine
Clonazepam
Clorazepate
Clozapine (31%)
Delavirdine
Dexmedetomidine
Diazepam
Diazoxide
Dimercaprol
Echinacea
Edrophonium (>10%)
Eletriptan
Estazolam
Ethionamide
Etodolac
Fluoxetine
Fluphenazine
Flurazepam
Fluvoxamine
Frovatriptan
Gabapentin
Gadodiamide

Galantamine
Gentamicin
Guanabenz
Guanethidine
Guanfacine
Haloperidol
Ibuprofen
Ifosfamide
Imatinib
Imipenem/Cilastatin
Indomethacin
Interferon alfa-2A
Interferon beta-1B
Irinotecan
Kanamycin
Ketamine
Ketoprofen
Lamotrigine
Levobetaxolol
Levobunolol
Levodopa
Lithium
Loratadine
Lorazepam
Maprotiline
Mefenamic acid
Mesoridazine
Methantheline
Methoxyflurane
Methohexital
Methylphenidate
Metipranolol
Metolazone
Midazolam
Mirtazapine
Modafinil
Molindone
Nabumetone
Naproxen
Naratriptan
Nefazodone
Neomycin
Nicotine (>10%)
Olanzapine

Ondansetron
Oxaprozin
Oxazepam
Oxybutynin
Pancuronium
Pantoprazole
Paroxetine
Pentoxifylline
Perphenazine
Phenindamine
Physostigmine (>10%)
Pilocarpine
Pimozide (14%)
Piroxicam
Potassium iodide
Pramipexole
Prazepam
Prochlorperazine
Promazine
Promethazine
Propofol
Quazepam
Quetiapine
Ramipril
Rapacuronium
Reserpine
Risperidone
Rivastigmine
Ropinirole
Selenium
Sertraline
Sodium oxybate
Succinylcholine
Tacrine
Temazepam
Thiothixene
Tiagabine
Tinidazole
Tobramycin
Tolcapone
Topiramate
Trazodone
Triazolam
Trovafloxacin

Valproic acid
Venlafaxine
Vigabatrin
Zaleplon (<1%)
Ziprasidone

STOMATITIS

Carmustine
Chlorhexidine
Chloroquine
Cidofovir
Clarithromycin
Clofibrate
Cloxacillin
Co-Trimoxazole
Corticosteroids
Cyclobenzaprine
Cyclophosphamide (10%)
Cyclosporine
Dacarbazine
Daptomycin
Daunorubicin (>10%)
Delavirdine
Desipramine
Diflunisal
Docetaxel (5–42%)
Doxepin
Doxorubicin (>10%)
Eletriptan
Enoxacin
Epirubicin
Ethionamide
Etidronate
Etodolac
Etoposide
Fenoprofen
Floxuridine
Fludarabine (>10%)
Fluorouracil (>10%)
Fluoxetine
Fluoxymesterone
Flurbiprofen
Fluvoxamine
Foscarnet

Gabapentin
Gatifloxacin
Gemcitabine (11%)
Gemtuzumab (25–32%)
Gentamicin
Ginkgo biloba
Glatiramer
Gold (>10%)
Granulocyte colony-stimulating factor
(GCSF) (>10%)
Griseofulvin
Hydroxychloroquine
Hydroxyurea (>10%)
Ibuprofen
Idarubicin (11%)
Ifosfamide
Imatinib
Imipramine
Indomethacin
Interferon alfa-2A
Ipratropium
Irinotecan (<14%)
Ketoprofen
Ketorolac
Lamivudine
Lamotrigine
Lansoprazole
Leflunomide
Levamisole
Levofloxacin
Lidocaine
Lincomycin
Lithium
Lomefloxacin
Lomustine
Loratadine
Lovastatin
Maprotiline
Meclofenamate
Mefenamic acid
Melphalan
Mephenytoin
Meprobamate
Mercaptopurine

Methenamine
Methicillin
Methotrexate
Methyltestosterone
Metronidazole
Mezlocillin
Mirtazapine
Mitomycin (>10%)
Mitoxantrone
Moxifloxacin
Mupirocin
Nabumetone
Nafcillin
Naproxen
Nefazodone
Nevirapine
Nicotine
Norfloxacin
Nortriptyline
Ofloxacin
Olsalazine
Oxacillin
Oxaliplatin (14%)
Oxaprozin
Oxcarbazepine
Paclitaxel (2–39%)
Pamidronate
Pantoprazole
Paroxetine
Pegfilgrastim
Pemetrexed (2–28%)
Penicillamine
Pentostatin (>10%)
Peppermint
Phenindamine
Phenytoin
Pilocarpine
Piperacillin
Piroxicam
Plicamycin (>10%)
Pravastatin
Procarbazine (>10%)
Propolis
Protriptyline

Pyrilamine
Quetiapine
Quinine
Quinupristin/Dalfopristin
Rabeprazole
Rifampin
Rimantadine
Risperidone
Ropinirole
Zalcitabine
Zaleplon (<1%)
Zonisamide (<1%)

STOMATODYNIA
Anisindione
Bacampicillin
Benztropine
Biperiden
Carbenicillin
Erythromycin
Ethionamide
Floxuridine
Garlic
Lithium
Methicillin
Mezlocillin
Nafcillin
Oxacillin
Piperacillin
Potassium iodide

STROKE
Abciximab (<1%)
Acitretin (<1%)
Agalsidase
Allopurinol IV
Atenolol
Celecoxib
Bortezomib
Clozapine
Dofetilide
Doxazosin
Ethacrynic acid
Glatiramer

Interferon alfa-2A
Irbesartan
Isotretinoin
Isradipine
Lamotrigine
Letrozole
Losartan
Nisoldipine
Perindopril
Quinapril
Ramipril
Risperidone
Rizatriptan
Smallpox vaccine
Tamoxifen
Ziprasidone

SYNCOPE

Abarelix
Acamprosate
Alemtuzumab
Alfuzosin (<1%)
Almotriptan (<1%)
Alprazolam (3–4%)
Amlodipine
Amoxapine
Anagrelide
Azithromycin
Baclofen
Benazepril
Bepridil
Bevacizumab
Bexarotene
Bicalutamide
Bivalirudin
Botulinum toxin (a & b)
Bretylium
Bromocriptine
Bupropion
Cabergoline
Capecitabine
Captopril
Carbamazepine
Carbinoxamine

Carisoprodol
Carteolol
Carvedilol
Cefpodoxime
Celecoxib
Cetirizine
Cevimeline
Chlorpromazine
Ciprofloxacin
Citalopram
Clonidine
Clopidogrel
Clozapine
Cyclobenzaprine
Cytarabine
Daptomycin
Darbepoetin alfa
Delavirdine
Denileukin
Dextroamphetamine
Dicloxacillin
Dicumarol
Dicyclomine
Diethylpropion
Diflunisal
Digoxin
Diltiazem
Dinoprostone
Dipyridamole
Disopyramide
Dobutamine
Docetaxel
Dofetilide
Domperidone
Donepezil
Doxazosin
Dronabinol
Edrophonium
Efavirenz
Enalapril
Enflurane
Enoxaparin
Entacapone
Epoetin alfa

Eprosartan
Ertapenem
Erythromycin
Estrogens
Ethchlorvynol
Etodolac
Felodipine
Fentanyl
Flecainide
Fluoxetine
Fluphenazine
Flurbiprofen
Flutamide
Foscarnet
Fosinopril
Fosphenytoin
Frovatriptan
Fulvestrant
Gadodiamide
Galantamine
Gatifloxacin
Gemfibrozil
Gemtuzumab
Glatiramer
Glipizide
Granisetron
Granulocyte colony-stimulating factor (GCSF)
Guanadrel
Guanethidine
Guanfacine
Haloperidol
Halothane
Hepatitis B vaccine
Hyaluronic acid
Hydroxyurea
Hydroxyzine
Hyoscyamine
Ibandronate
Ibritumomab
Ibuprofen
Ifosfamide
Imatinib (11–13%)
Imiglucerase

Imipenem/Cilastatin
Indomethacin
Interferon alfa-2A
Interferon beta-1B
Irbesartan
Irinotecan
Isosorbide dinitrate
Isosorbide mononitrate
Isoxsuprine
Ketamine
Labetalol
Laronidase
Leflunomide
Letrozole
Leuprolide
Levalbuterol
Levodopa
Levofloxacin
Lithium
Lomefloxacin
Loratadine
Losartan
Loxapine
Maprotiline
Medroxyprogesterone
Meloxicam
Mepenzolate
Mephenytoin
Mephobarbital
Meprobamate
Mesoridazine
Metaxalone
Methamphetamine
Methantheline
Methicillin
Methocarbamol
Methohexital
Methoxyflurane
Metolazone
Metoprolol
Mexiletine
Mezlocillin
Midodrine
Mifepristone

Moexipril
Moricizine
Moxifloxacin
Nabumetone
Nadolol
Nafcillin
Naproxen
Naratriptan
Natalizumab
Nefazodone
Nelfinavir
Nesiritide
Niacin
Nicardipine
Nifedipine
Nisoldipine
Nitisinone
Nitroglycerin
Norfloxacin
Ofloxacin
Orphenadrine
Oxaprozin
Oxcarbazepine
Oxybutynin
Oxycodone
Palonosetron
Pamidronate
Pantoprazole
Paroxetine
Penbutolol
Penicillins
Pentagastrin
Pentazocine
Pentobarbital
Pergolide
Perindopril
Perphenazine
Phendimetrazine
Phenindamine
Phenobarbital
Phenoxybenzamine
Phentermine
Phenytoin
Phytonadione

Pilocarpine
Pimozide
Pindolol
Piperacillin
Piroxicam
Pramipexole
Prazepam
Prazosin
Procarbazine
Prochlorperazine
Promazine
Promethazine
Propantheline
Propofol
Propoxyphene
Propranolol
Quazepam
Quetiapine
Quinapril
Quinethazone
Quinidine
Quinine
Quinupristin/Dalfopristin
Rabeprazole
Ramipril
Reteplase
Ritonavir
Rivastigmine
Rizatriptan
Ropinirole (12%)
Rosuvastatin
Sildenafil
Sirolimus
Streptokinase
Tegaserod
Telithromycin
Telmisartan
Terazosin
Teriparatide
Thioguanine
Timolol
Tinidazole
Tinzaparin
Tizanidine

Trandolapril
Travoprost
Trazodone
Treprostinil
Trichlormethiazide
Vardenafil
Vasopressin
Verapamil
Zanamivir
Zoledronic acid
Zolmitriptan

TARDIVE DYSKINESIA

Amitriptyline
Amoxapine
Aripiprazole
Chlorpheniramine
Chlorpromazine
Clozapine
Doxepin
Droperidol
Ethotoin
Fluphenazine
Haloperidol (37%)
Loxapine
Mesoridazine
Metoclopramide
Molindone
Olanzapine
Oxacillin
Palivizumab
Perphenazine
Prochlorperazine
Promazine
Promethazine
Quetiapine
Risperidone
Ziprasidone

TINNITUS

Alprazolam (6.6%)
Amiloride
Aminocaproic acid
Amitriptyline

Amlodipine
Amoxapine
Amphotericin B
Anagrelide
Anthrax vaccine
Aprepitant
Aripiprazole
Arsenic
Artemisia
Aspirin
Azithromycin
Aztreonam
Baclofen
Balsalazide
Benazepril
Benztropine
Bepridil
Betaxolol
Bismuth
Bisoprolol
Botulinum toxin (a & b)
Calcitonin
Capreomycin
Carbamazepine
Carisoprodol
Carteolol
Carvedilol
Cefpodoxime
Celecoxib
Cevimeline
Chlordiazepoxide (1–10%)
Chloroquine
Chlorpheniramine
Cholestyramine
Cinoxacin
Ciprofloxacin
Citalopram
Clarithromycin
Clemastine
Co-Trimoxazole
Codeine
Cyclobenzaprine
Cyclosporine
Deferoxamine

Demeclocycline
Desipramine
Devil's claw
Diazoxide
Diclofenac
Diflunisal
Diltiazem
Dimenhydrinate
Diphenhydramine
Dipyridamole
Doxazosin
Doxepin
Dronabinol
Efavirenz
Eletriptan
Enalapril
Enoxacin
Eprosartan
Erythromycin
Escitalopram
Esomeprazole
Estramustine
Estrogens
Etanercept
Ethacrynic acid
Etodolac
Famotidine
Felodipine
Fenoprofen
Flecainide
Flumazenil
Fluoxetine
Flurazepam
Flurbiprofen
Foscarnet
Fosinopril
Fosphenytoin
Frovatriptan
Furosemide
Gabapentin
Gadodiamide
Gatifloxacin
Gentamicin
Glatiramer

Guanfacine
Guarana
Hepatitis B vaccine
Hydrocodone
Hydroxychloroquine
Hydroxyzine
Ibuprofen
Imipenem/Cilastatin
Imipramine
Indomethacin
Interferon alfa-2A
Isoniazid
Isotretinoin
Isradipine
Itraconazole
Ketoconazole
Ketoprofen
Ketorolac
Labetalol
Lansoprazole
Levobetaxolol
Levobunolol
Levobupivacaine
Levofloxacin
Lidocaine
Lincomycin
Lisinopril
Lithium
Lomefloxacin
Loratadine
Maprotiline
Mechlorethamine
Meclofenamate
Mefenamic acid
Mefloquine
Meloxicam
Memantine
Meperidine
Mephenytoin
Mesalamine
Methadone
Methazolamide
Methotrexate
Metipranolol

Metolazone
Metoprolol
Mexiletine
Minocycline
Misoprostol
Moexipril
Moricizine
Morphine
Moxifloxacin
Mycophenolate
Nabumetone
Nadolol
Nalbuphine
Naltrexone
Naproxen
Nefazodone
Nicardipine
Nicotine
Nifedipine
Nisoldipine
Nizatidine
Norfloxacin
Nortriptyline
Ofloxacin
Olsalazine
Omeprazole
Oxaprozin
Oxycodone
Paclitaxel
Palivizumab
Palonosetron
Pantoprazole
Paroxetine
Penbutolol
Penicillamine
Pentazocine
Pentosan
Pentostatin
Pergolide
Perindopril
Perphenazine
Phenindamine
Phenytoin
Pilocarpine

Pindolol
Piperacillin
Piroxicam
Prazosin
Prochlorperazine
Promazine
Promethazine
Propantheline
Propofol
Propoxyphene
Protriptyline
Pseudoephedrine
Pyrazinamide
Pyrimethamine
Quinethazone
Quinidine
Quinine
Ramipril
Ranitidine
Risedronate
Rizatriptan
Ropinirole
Salsalate
Sirolimus
Sodium oxybate
Streptokinase
Sulfadiazine
Sulindac
Thiabendazole
Tinzaparin
Tolmetin
Torsemide
Travoprost
Trazodone
Trimipramine
Vancomycin
Zalcitabine
Zolpidem

TREMOR
Acamprosate
Acyclovir
Acamprosate
Acyclovir

Adalimumab (5%)
Albuterol
Alemtuzumab (7%)
Allopurinol IV
Almotriptan
Alosetron
Alprazolam (4–10%)
Altretamine (<1%)
Amantadine
Amikacin (<1%)
Amiloride
Aminophylline
Amiodarone
Amitriptyline
Amlodipine
Amoxapine
Amphotericin B
Anthrax vaccine
Arbutamine
Aripiprazole
Asparaginase
Atomoxetine
Atropine sulfate
Baclofen
Balsalazide
Basiliximab
Benzonatate
Benzphetamine
Bepridil
Bismuth
Black cohosh
Botulinum toxin (a & b)
Buclizine
Bupropion (>10%)
Cabergoline
Caffeine
Capecitabine
Carbamazepine
Carisoprodol
Caspofungin
Cefaclor
Cetirizine
Cevimeline (<10%)
Chlorambucil

Chlordiazepoxide (1–10%)
Chlorpromazine
Chlorzoxazone
Ciprofloxacin
Citalopram
Clarithromycin
Clofarabine (10%)
Clomipramine (>10%)
Clonazepam (>10%)
Clonidine
Clorazepate
Clozapine
Co-trimoxazole
Cocaine
Codeine
Cyclobenzaprine
Cyclosporine (12–55%)
Daclizumab
Dantrolene
Dapsone
Desipramine
Diazepam
Diazoxide
Dicyclomine
Diethylpropion
Diflunisal
Diltiazem
Dimenhydrinate
Dinoprostone
Diphenhydramine
Dipyridamole
Dirithromycin
Domperidone
Donepezil
Doxepin
Duloxetine
Efavirenz
Eletriptan
Enflurane
Enoxacin
Entacapone
Ephedra
Ephedrine
Eprosartan

Ertapenem
Escitalopram
Estrogens
Ethchlorvynol
Ethotoin
Etodolac
Flecainide
Felbamate
Fludarabine
Flumazenil
Fluoxetine (3–13%)
Fluphenazine
Flurazepam
Flurbiprofen
Fluvastatin
Fluvoxamine
Formoterol
Fosinopril
Fosphenytoin
Frovatriptan
Gabapentin
Gadodiamide
Galantamine
Ganciclovir
Gatifloxacin
Gemifloxacin
Gemtuzumab
Gentamicin
Glatiramer
Glipizide
Glycopyrrolate
Guanadrel
Haloperidol
Halothane
Hydralazine
Hydrocodone
Hydroxyzine
Ibandronate
Ibuprofen
Imipenem/Cilastatin
Imipramine
Immune globulin IV
Indomethacin
Insulin

Interferon alfa-2A
Interferon beta-1A
Interferon beta-1B
Ipratropium
Irbesartan
Isoetharine
Isoflurane
Isoproterenol
Ivermectin
Kanamycin (<1%)
Ketamine (>10%)
Ketoconazole
Ketoprofen
Lamotrigine
Lansoprazole
Levalbuterol
Levetiracetam
Levobupivacaine
Levodopa
Levofloxacin
Levothyroxine
Lidocaine
Liothyronine
Lisinopril
Lithium
Lomefloxacin
Loratadine
Lorazepam
Losartan
Loxapine
Maprotiline
Mazindol
MDMA
Mecamylamine
Meclizine
Meclofenamate
Mefenamic acid
Mefloquine
Meloxicam
Meperidine
Mephenytoin
Mesoridazine
Metaxalone
Methadone

Methamphetamine
Methazolamide
Methocarbamol
Methohexital (>10%)
Methoxyflurane (>10%)
Mexiletine (13%)
Miglustat (30%)
Mirtazapine
Misoprostol
Mitotane
Modafinil
Molindone
Monosodium glutamate
Morphine
Moxifloxacin
Mycophenolate (24–34%)
Nabumetone
Nalbuphine
Nalidixic acid
Naloxone
Naltrexone
Naproxen
Natalizumab
Nedocromil
Nefazodone
Nelfinavir
Neomycin
Nesiritide
Nicotine
Nifedipine
Nisoldipine
Norfloxacin
Nortriptyline
Ofloxacin
Olanzapine
Omeprazole
Oral contraceptives
Orphenadrine
Oxaprozin
Oxazepam
Oxcarbazepine (3–16%)
Oxycodone
Palonosetron
Pamidronate

Pantoprazole
Paroxetine
Pemoline
Pentamidine
Pentazocine
Pentoxifylline
Pergolide
Perindopril
Perphenazine
Phendimetrazine
Phenelzine
Phenindamine
Phentermine
Phenylephrine
Phenylpropanolamine
Phenytoin
Pilocarpine
Pimozide
Pirbuterol
Piroxicam
Pravastatin
Prazepam
Procainamide
Procarbazine (>10%)
Prochlorperazine
Procyclidine
Promazine
Promethazine
Propafenone
Propofol (>10%)
Propoxyphene
Protriptyline
Pseudoephedrine
Quetiapine
Quinapril
Quinethazone
Quinidine
Quinine
Quinupristin/dalfopristin
Risperidone (14%)
Rabeprazole
Ramipril
Reserpine
Risperidone

Ritodrine (>10%)
Rivastigmine
Rizatriptan
Ropinirole
Rosiglitazone
Salmeterol
Selegiline
Selenium
Sertraline
Sirolimus
Sodium oxybate
Sparfloxacin
Streptomycin
Sulfadoxine
Sulfamethoxazole
Tacrine
Tacrolimus
Tea tree
Telithromycin
Temazepam
Temozolomide
Tenofovir
Terbutaline
Thalidomide
Thioridazine
Thiopental
Thioridazine
Thiothixene
Tiagabine
Tinidazole
Tizanidine
Tobramycin
Tocainide
Topiramate
Tramadol
Tranylcypromine
Trazodone
Tretinoin
Triazolam
Trifluoperazine
Trimethoprim
Trimipramine
Tripelennamine
Trazodone

Trimethobenzamide
Trimetrexate
Trimipramine
Triprolidine
Valdecoxib
Valerian
Valproic acid
Vasopressin
Venlafaxine
Vigabatrin
Voriconazole
Zalcitabine
Zaleplon (1–10%)
Zidovudine
Ziprasidone (<1%)
Zolpidem (<1%)
Zonisamide (<1%)

TWITCHING
Acamprosate
Allopurinol IV
Alprazolam (8%)
Arbutamine
Aripiprazole
Atazanavir
Bupropion
Cabergoline
Caffeine
Carbachol (eyelids)
Carbamazepine
Carbinoxamine
Cetirizine
Chlorambucil
Citalopram
Clonazepam
Cycloserine
Dextroamphetamine
Dicyclomine
Dolasetron
Eletriptan
Entacapone
Escitalopram
Flecainide
Fluoxetine

Flurbiprofen
Fluvoxamine
Fosphenytoin
Gabapentin
Gemtuzumab
Gentamicin
Glycopyrrolate
Horse chestnut (bark, flower, leaf, seed)
Ketoprofen
Lamotrigine
Levodopa
Lidocaine
Lithium
Mefenamic acid
Mephenytoin
Methamphetamine
Mitotane
Naltrexone
Nefazodone
Olanzapine
Pemoline
Phenelzine
Phenytoin
Physostigmine
Pramipexole
Propofol
Quetiapine
Rabeprazole
Rasburicase
Reteplase
Risperidone
Ropinirole
Streptokinase
Thiopental
Tolcapone
Tranylcypromine
Valdecoxib
Voriconazole
Zalcitabine
Ziprasidone
Zoledronic acid
Zolmitriptan (<1%)

VISION BLURRED
Baclofen
Scopolamine
Sertraline
Sildenafil
Simvastatin
Sirolimus
Sodium oxybate
Solifenacin
Somatropin
Streptokinase
Streptomycin
Sumatriptan
Tartrazine
Telithromycin
Temazepam
Terazosin
Thioridazine
Thiothixene
Tiagabine
Tinzaparin
Tiotropium
Tizanidine
Tolazamide
Tolbutamide
Tolterodine
Topiramate
Toremifene
Tramadol
Tranylcypromine
Travoprost
Trazodone
Treprostinil
Triazolam
Trifluoperazine
Trihexyphenidyl
Trimeprazine
Trimethobenzamide
Trimipramine
Triprolidine
Trovafloxacin
Valdecoxib
Valganciclovir
Vardenafil

Venlafaxine
Vidarabine
Vigabatrin
Voriconazole
Zoledronic acid

WEIGHT CHANGE
Cabergoline
Carvedilol (11%)
Cefditoren
Cevimeline
Chlordiazepoxide (>10%)
Chlorpromazine
Citalopram
Clofazimine
Clofibrate
Clomipramine (>10%)
Clozapine (>10%)
Corticosteroids
Cyclosporine
Daptomycin
Darbepoetin alfa
Denileukin (14%)
Desipramine
Diazoxide
Diethylstilbestrol
Dihydrotachysterol
Dimenhydrinate
Diphenhydramine
Disopyramide
Dofetilide
Doxepin
Doxercalciferol
Droperidol
Efavirenz
Enflurane
Enfuvirtide
Epoetin alfa
Ergocalciferol
Ertapenem
Estrogens
Etanercept
Ethionamide
Etodolac

Fenofibrate
Fludarabine
Fluoxetine
Fluoxymesterone
Fluphenazine
Flurbiprofen
Fluvoxamine
Fosamprenavir
Fosphenytoin
Fulvestrant
Galantamine
Ganirelix
Gefitinib
Glatiramer
Glimepiride
Glipizide
Glyburide
Goserelin
Halothane
Hydroxychloroquine
Ibritumomab
Ibuprofen
Imipramine
Indapamide
Indinavir
Indomethacin
Insulin
Interferon alfa-2A
Interferon beta-1A
Interferon beta-1B
Irinotecan
Isoflurane
Isotretinoin
Itraconazole
Ketamine
Ketoconazole
Lamotrigine
Letrozole
Leuprolide
Levalbuterol
Levodopa
Liothyronine
Lithium
Loratadine

Lorazepam
Losartan
Maprotiline
Meclizine
Medroxyprogesterone
Mefloquine
Meloxicam
Memantine
Mephenytoin
Mesoridazine
Metformin
Methadone
Methamphetamine
Methimazole
Methohexital
Methoxyflurane
Methyltestosterone
Methysergide
Miglustat (39–67%)
Minoxidil
Mirtazapine (12%)
Misoprostol
Mitoxantrone
Molindone
Morphine
Nabumetone
Nafarelin
Nalbuphine
Naltrexone
Naproxen
Nateglinide
Nelfinavir
Nitazoxanide
Nortriptyline
Ofloxacin
Olanzapine
Olmesartan
Oxazepam
Oxybutynin
Palonosetron
Paramethadione
Paroxetine
Peginterferon alfa-2B (11%)
Pegvisomant

Pemetrexed
Pemoline
Pentostatin
Perphenazine
Phenazopyridine
Phenelzine
Pioglitazone (>10%)
Pramipexole
Prazepam
Probenecid
Prochlorperazine
Promazine
Promethazine
Propofol
Propylthiouracil
Protriptyline
Quetiapine
Raloxifene
Rasburicase
Reteplase
Rituximab
Rivastigmine
Ropinirole
Sargramostin
Sertraline
Sibutramine
Sirolimus
Spironolactone
Stavudine
Streptokinase
Thioguanine
Thioridazine
Thiotepa
Thiothixene
Timolol
Tinidazole
Tizanidine
Topiramate
Tranylcypromine
Trazodone
Trifluoperazine
Trimipramine
Urofollitropin
Valdecoxib

Vasopressin
Vigabatrin
Voriconazole
Zidovudine
Zoledronic acid

XANTHOPSIA

Bendroflumethiazide
Chlorothiazide
Tadalafil
Thiabendazole
Vigabatrin

YAWNING

Apomorphine
Citalopram
Clomipramine
Fluoxetine
Fluvoxamine
Paroxetine
Pilocarpine
Ropinirole

T - #0155 - 071024 - C0 - 178/127/16 - PB - 9780415383806 - Gloss Lamination